Freedom From Neck & Back Pain

Learn to Live an Active Life

Without Fear of Pain

By Dr. Tamer Issa

Copyright © 2022 Tamer Issa. All rights reserved.

This publication is licensed to the individual reader only. Duplication or distribution by any means, including email, disk, photocopy, and recording, to a person other than the original purchaser, is a violation of international copyright law.

Publisher: Tamer Issa, Issa Physical Therapy & Wellness, P.O. Box 114 Ashton, MD 20861

While they have made every effort to verify the information here, neither the author nor the publisher assumes any responsibility for errors in, omissions from, or a different interpretation of the subject matter. This information may be subject to varying laws and practices in other areas, states, and countries. The reader assumes all responsibility for the use of the information. Any implication of the information herein is the reader's own risk. Any individual with a specific health problem or who is taking medication should seek advice from their personal physician or healthcare provider before starting any self-care program, especially one that includes a change in diet or levels of exercise.

The purpose of this book is to inform and educate. No individual should use the information in this book for self-diagnosis, treatment, or as justification for accepting or declining any medical therapy for any health problem or disease. No individual is discouraged from seeking professional medical advice and treatment. This book is not supplying medical advice.

The author and publisher shall in no event be held liable to any party for any damages arising directly or indirectly from any use of this material. Every effort has been made to represent our products and services and their potential accurately.

Illustrations by Viktorija Gordejeva

Editing by David Walker

Dedication

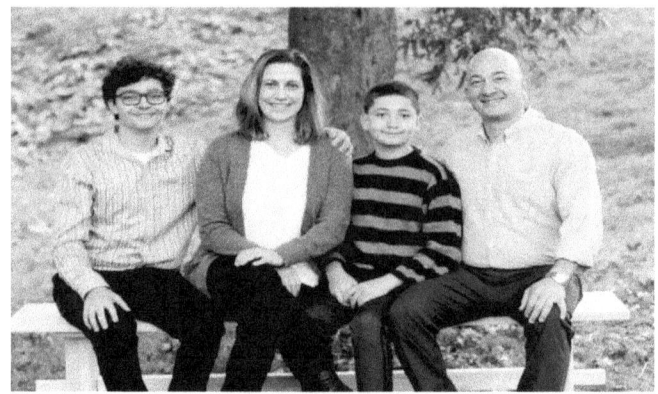

To my wife, Cheryl-

Thank you for your unwavering support and love. Without it, this book and many of my other aspirations in life wouldn't have been possible. Love always!

To my boys Jacob and Ben-

Thank you for keeping me young at heart. You are both incredible spirits, and I'm blessed to be your dad. I look forward to watching your unique gifts and talents blossom in this life. Always remember that anything is possible! Love you both, Papa!

To my mom, Souzan, and my dad, Salah-

Words aren't enough to express my gratitude to you both. Thank you for the sacrifices you made coming to a foreign country to build a life for your future family that allowed your kids opportunities that we may have never had. Thank you for setting an excellent example of loving and supportive parents. Dad, I know you would have been very proud of this book!

Acknowledgments

To my past teachers and mentors, including Ricardo Van Ravensberg and the professors at the Hogeschool Enschede in the Netherlands, Jan Dommerholt, Dr. Robert Gerwin, and the late Peter Huijbregts. Thank you for your inspiration and guidance.

Thank you to my special friend and personal trainer, Pasquale "Lino" Silvestre. You introduced me to the world of European Posturology and the Raggi Method. My sessions with you on the Pancafit table using the Raggi Method and the functional training you provided me were instrumental in my interest and understanding of postural rebalancing, the role of fascia, the Dynamic Neuromuscular Stabilization (DNS) method, and functional stability and strength. Most importantly, thank you for your friendship. Ciao!

Thank you to Prof. Pavel Kolář, Dr. Alena Kobesova, and the Dynamic Neuromuscular Stabilization (DNS) instructors at the Rehabilitation Prague School in the Czech Republic and the United States. Over the years, learning the DNS method has been one of the best experiences of my personal life and professional career. It has deepened my understanding of human development, postural expression, and movement behavior. Learning and utilizing the DNS method has made a significant positive impact on both my own and my patients' physical limitations.

Thank you to Prof. Daniele Raggi and the Raggi Method Pancafit instructors from Milan, Italy. Learning the Raggi Method using the

Pancafit bench has profoundly affected my understanding of Posturology and the global approach to postural rebalancing. Thank you for taking the time to come to the US and teach some American physical therapists this extraordinary approach.

Thank you to all my past and current clients. You have contributed to this book in some way or another. I learned and gained something from each of you in our sessions together. All the education, training, and experience gained over the years have been in the pursuit of helping improve your optimal physical health and well-being.

A big thank you to Paul Gough and his team! Not only have you helped my physical therapy business succeed, but you have had a profound positive effect on my personal life. Thanks for inspiring me to chase my dreams and write this book.

To my editor, David Walker. Thanks for all your work on editing the book and allowing for it to be more understandable and impactful for people.

To all who read this book. Thank you for taking the time to read it. Please pass it along to someone you think could be helped by it.

Testimonials

"Working with Tamer to learn and incorporate dynamic neuromuscular stabilization techniques into my training was game-changing as a runner and triathlete. These techniques not only enabled me to train and compete without injury for the past three years but also helped me to continue running throughout my entire 2nd pregnancy, to resume running post-delivery safely, and to train for and compete in my first 50k ultramarathon 17 months postpartum, placing 1st among women."

Kristin (Age 41)

Bethesda, MD

"I am a Professional Golf Instructor and have dealt with back and shoulder pain for almost half my life! Tamer's guidance and use of the breathing exercises to stabilize my core significantly improved me while other physical therapists failed. I have become more functional and can now play golf pain-free. Tamer has the experience, skill, and knowledge to keep me doing what I love. Not only is he a great PT, but he is hands down one of the kindest and caring individuals I know."

Kevin (Age 36)

PGA Master Professional

Mt. Airy, MD

"I can't say enough about my results on my posture using the Pancafit table! I had chronic pain from severe scoliosis. Using breathing and core exercises helped me develop core muscles I never had. Then the Pancafit work helped my soft tissue to be more resilient during the activities in my daily life. Combined with my stretching, exercise routines, and physical therapy, it has allowed me to be pain-free most of the time. It's a technique that will continue to serve me as I age, keeping me as active and pain-free as possible."

Carol (Age 68)

Kensington, MD

"The postural, breathing, and stability strategies outlined by Tamer have become a foundational pillar upon which I have built a balanced healthy lifestyle and achieved improved, injury-free, athletic performance."

Dan (Age 46)

Ashton, MD

"I love to hike, but over the years, I've been hampered by pain, tendonitis, and weakness due partly to hyper-mobility and lax muscles. Recovery would take many months and be so frustrating. Previous physical therapy experiences sometimes actually made me worse. My experience with the posture rebalancing approach on the Pancafit bench and the DNS postural stability core work has allowed me to avoid pain and remain active without long periods of injury and recovery."

Elise (Age 64)

Silver Spring, MD

"I never thought that my breathing and posture affected my health as much as they did until working with Dr. Tamer. By changing my breathing and learning to engage my core, I was able to work through my shoulder injury and come back stronger and faster."

Ella (Age 14)

Rockville, MD

"When I first came to Tamer, my sciatica was so bad that I often had difficulty getting out of bed in the morning. I had tried traditional physical therapy and osteopathic treatment, but nothing was successful. Posture balancing, dry needling, and breathing exercises brought almost immediate relief. My exercise plan has strengthened my core. I have seen a marked improvement in my balance; I have more stamina and feel better than I have in years. I am committed to this approach."

Ellen (Age 74)

Washington, DC

"When I came to Dr. Issa, I was coming off a hard Cross-Country season and two muscular injuries in my lower legs. I was in a tremendous amount of pain, but with the help of Dr. Issa, we were able to heal the injuries. As my lower legs recovered from their injuries, we looked to correct the underlying problems in my hips and spine to help decrease the chances of another injury. Through our weekly (then monthly) visits, we worked on hip and core strengthening through exercises and dry needling. These exercises helped me greatly prepare for my spring track season and helped me achieve new personal records I would never have thought possible."

Julien (Age 18)

Potomac, MD

"Dr. Issa treated my then-teenage son for approximately two years on issues of residual neurologic impairment resulting from a prenatal stroke. My son improved significantly during that time with pain relief, postural stability and balance, core strength, muscle balance, correcting maladaptive movement patterns, and improving gait. He has maintained these gains through the training program that Tamer developed for him. He is now 21 years old, remains pain-free, and thrives physically and psychologically because of increased confidence and self-esteem."

Terri (Mother)

Rockville, MD

"Struggling with myofascial pain, Tamer used his toolkit of dry-needling and manual stretching to relieve my discomfort. That alone made him a valuable asset. He then taught me to lock down my core muscles using movements modeled after babies, which enabled me to develop a comprehensive program to maintain upper and lower body strength and avoid glitches. That made Tamer an invaluable asset. Read, learn, and practice."

Bruce (Age 70)

Silver Spring, MD

CONTENTS

Introduction 13

CHAPTER 1
Why Everything You Know About the "Core" Is Wrong 21

CHAPTER 2
Mistakes People Make in Addressing Chronic Neck & Back Pain 39

CHAPTER 3
My Personal Experience with Chronic Neck & Back Pain 62

CHAPTER 4
What Causes Spinal Instability 83

CHPATER 5
Posture & Postural Alignment 108

CHAPTER 6
Breathing 136

CHAPTER 7
Activating the Core 180

CHAPTER 8
Postural Stability in Everyday Life 224

CHAPTER 9
Getting Additional Help 258

CHAPTER 10
Moving Forward 272

Resources 276

About the Author 277

Introduction

I know of no more encouraging fact than the unquestionable ability of man to elevate his life by conscious endeavor.

Henry David Thoreau

That quote by Thoreau is one of my all-time favorites. This book was born out of such an endeavor, and I hope it will elevate the life of everyone who reads it. Let me share how it came to be.

After graduating from Penn State University in 1995 with a bachelor's degree in Exercise & Sport Science, I moved back home with my parents. I started working as a Physical Therapy Aide at Bryn Mawr Rehab in Paoli, PA. Bryn Mawr Rehab is one of Pennsylvania's most comprehensive rehabilitation centers, specializing in inpatient and outpatient physical medicine and rehabilitation for spinal cord injuries, traumatic brain injuries, strokes, amputees, neurologic, and orthopedic conditions. I witnessed every possible specialty in physical therapy there, including aquatic therapy, work hardening, driver rehab, horticultural therapy, hippotherapy (benefits from riding horses), and more. It was a remarkable place, and the therapists and patients I interacted with profoundly affected me. My plan at the time was to attend a physical therapy graduate program. That year at Bryn Mawr Rehab confirmed that physical therapy was my calling.

One of my physical therapist friends clued me in on a physical therapy program in Holland for American students, taught in English. I didn't know how the Dutch physical therapy programs stacked against other countries. Still, she assured me they were excellent and that learning physical therapy from a different perspective would serve me well when I returned to work in the States. I investigated the program and discovered that the Dutch program was the first foreign program accredited by the American Physical Therapy Association. I spoke to my parents about it, and they supported my decision to apply. Two weeks later, I had an interview in Boston. One month after that, I was accepted. Three months later, I was in Holland for two years!

Those two years I spent in Holland was the best thing that ever happened to me (until getting married and having kids, of course!). Living abroad in Europe was a fantastic coming-of-age experience for me. Besides the obvious benefits of traveling Europe in my free time, I received a world-class education in physical therapy. That education set the foundation for the therapist I am today.

I learned three major lessons in Holland that still influence my practice today. The first was the emphasis on hands-on therapy skills. We had massage therapy every semester of school. Some American physical therapy programs only have one semester of soft tissue work; others have none. We also learned how to use our hands to mobilize joints and strengthen muscles without equipment. All that hands-on practice developed the touch I think every therapist needs to evaluate and treat effectively.

The second was a holistic approach to care. We had several courses in psychology and were taught the importance of patient-practitioner interactions. It was stressed that you are not just treating a physical problem (the knee, the shoulder, the back); you are treating a person with a physical problem. That's a big difference.

The third was the emphasis on clinical reasoning and critical thinking skills. This may sound obvious and necessary, but unfortunately, it often isn't a central component of many physical therapy programs in the US. We were expected to diagnose neuromusculoskeletal problems independently rather than rely on a physician's order or diagnosis. They taught us to think rather than follow a protocol-based approach. Our Dutch professors were tough on us, and I remember multiple times being challenged as to why we were doing what we were doing or thinking what we were thinking. I'm so grateful they did because it has served me well.

Once finished, I headed back to the States, ready to start my career. I was soon enlightened about the differences between the US and Netherlands physical therapy approaches. In my first year, I worked as an inpatient and outpatient physical therapist at a community hospital in Westminster, MD. Then I transferred to the outpatient orthopedic practice to pursue my interest there. I quit after a month. That was a rude awakening. I was seeing three patients an hour and felt I was doing a quarter of what I was capable of. Even as a new grad, I knew that was a bad sign. In Holland, all the therapy is carried out by the physical therapist in a one-on-one format with no treatment or help from a physical therapy assistant or aide.

I left and took a job at a pain management and rehabilitation medical practice in Bethesda, MD. Those five years set me on a path to becoming the exceptional therapist I was striving to be. I learned the importance and underappreciated contribution of muscle pain and dysfunction in neuromusculoskeletal conditions. I also learned dry needling early in my career, which set me apart. And under the mentorship of physical therapist Jan Dommerholt and Dr. Robert Gerwin, I was fortunate enough to start on a path of teaching continuing education courses, being published in journals and book chapters, and presenting at professional conferences. During those early years, I was passionate about developing my manual therapy skills through dozens of continuing education courses.

The skills I developed served me well, especially as I started my private practice in 2005. I decided to go out-of-network, except for Medicare, because I knew I wouldn't be able to provide the care I thought people deserved in an insurance-based model. My clinical reasoning and skills in manual therapy, dry needling, and functional exercises helped many people get out of pain and back to normal life over the years. I was grateful for that.

But there was a problem. People seemed to continually return to therapy after successful treatment, especially those suffering from recurrent, chronic neck and back issues. They would come back after three months, six months, a year, or more with similar complaints as to what brought them in, to begin with. There were plenty of plausible reasons for this, mostly centered around what the patient didn't do during their time away, not being consistent with their home exercise program, not changing their daily posture and body mechanics, and poor choices regarding exercise type and intensity. It's always easy to blame the patient, but I began to wonder whether I was doing something wrong.

In 2013, I gained clarity as to why people suffered from recurrent, chronic, nagging neck and back pain, and the ideas and concepts of this book were born. A lot of physical therapy interventions are aimed at treating symptoms. If you only treat the symptoms and don't address the underlying causes, symptoms are bound to recur. My clinical experience led me to discover that the underlying reasons for many chronic neck and back pain sufferers were spinal instability, postural imbalance, non-optimal breathing patterns, and poor body awareness.

A stable spine can meet the demands of the compressive, tensile, and shearing forces placed on it through gravity, bending, twisting, lifting, and other movement forces over time. An unstable spine does not meet these demands adequately, resulting in wear and tear of the spinal structures and leading to muscle imbalance compensations that further add to the forces on the spine. When the load exceeds the capacity, recurrent symptoms are inevitable until the underlying spinal stability is addressed.

It's not unusual for a physical therapist or other health and fitness professionals to recognize this phenomenon. A spine stabilization exercise program is a component of many therapists' approaches when addressing spinal pain and mobility problems. The lay person may understand this stability work as "core stability." The problem is that there continues to be an ongoing debate as to whether stability work is relevant in the prevalence of spine problems or the rehabilitation of spine problems. Scientific research has made strides in answering these questions. It has been clear to me that the coordination of muscles around our spine influences spinal stability, so improving this coordinated muscle activity can generate improved spinal stability. Our theories and approaches to alleviate spine problems through exercise have varied dramatically in the past 90 years, starting with the origin of Williams Flexion Exercises in the 1930s, which advocated abdominal strengthening, to the dynamic stabilization concepts in the 1990s, to the motor control concept of the late 1990s and 2000s, to the functional stability and strength concepts of the last 20 years.

This book will present a fundamental and practical approach to spinal stability mainly based on the Dynamic Neuromuscular Stabilization (DNS) concept developed by Pavel Kolář at the Rehabilitation Prague School. I have found this stabilization exercise system to be the most accurate, comprehensive, and effective approach. Throughout the book, I will use the terms "core stability," "postural stability," and "spinal stability" interchangeably to mean the same thing. Don't get hung up on the semantics. Focus on the bigger picture and how it relates to chronic neck and back spine pain. I will not only review a stabilization program that may help you, but I will also explain other factors that need to be addressed for optimal spinal stability, including postural alignment, optimal breathing patterns, and body awareness.

The book's first chapter starts with addressing some common misconceptions of the "core" that introduce you to what makes up our core stability, postural stability, or spinal stability. The second chapter will address common ways people deal with chronic neck and back issues and why those may not be solving the problem. The third chapter will describe my personal experience with chronic neck and back pain and how I came to learn of the clinical approach that I describe throughout the book. The fourth chapter covers the factors contributing to spinal instability and will answer one of the most common questions I get from people when they come to see me for neck and back pain: why do I have this problem? The fifth chapter covers the critical role that posture and postural alignment play. The sixth chapter covers dysfunctional versus optimal breathing patterns and how the diaphragm affects your posture and ability to stabilize your spine. The seventh chapter is an in-depth look at spinal stability, where it comes from, and how to improve it. The eighth chapter is a practical guide to improving your awareness of postural stability in everyday life. The ninth chapter reviews possible solutions and why you should consider physical therapy. The tenth chapter is a summary and guide to help you move forward in finding a solution to your chronic neck or back pain.

This book will challenge the cultural and medical norms of how we address chronic spine issues and how to engage your core. I aim to educate as many people as possible on the concepts in this book at the heart of chronic spinal problems and, most importantly, solutions that work in addressing them.

Whether you are suffering from a chronic neck or back problem, looking to prevent possible spinal issues, or a health or fitness professional who works with people with spinal problems, this book will have something for you. Additional resources can be found at: www.freedomfromneckandbackpain.com

Be Well,

Tamer

Dr. Tamer Issa, PT, DPT, OCS

Doctor of Physical Therapy

Issa Physical Therapy & Wellness

CHAPTER 1

Why Everything You Know About the "Core" Is Wrong

"The difficulty lies not so much in developing new ideas as in escaping from old ones."

John Maynard Keynes

Myth: The "Core" is Another Name for Your Abdominals, and It Needs Strengthening

Most people think your "core" is another name for your abdominals. Not true. Many think that you must have a strong body if you have strong abs. Also, false. But these misconceptions are why people who want to strengthen and protect their backs often work on their abs. Not only is it wrong, but it is often counterproductive and may exacerbate the problem. Most people need to learn to activate and control their core, not strengthen their abs.

So, what is your core?

The first definition in the Oxford dictionary is: **"the most important or central part of something."** This is a beautifully simple definition. It is as accurate of your body in its posture and ability to move as it is of an apple in its ability to grow or a power plant in its ability to electrify. Without the core, everything else would be useless. We'll come back to this idea later.

The dictionary's fourth definition is: **"the muscles of the lower back and stomach area which help you maintain balance, etc."** As a technical definition, this is true, but it doesn't tell the whole story.

The core comprises a group of muscles that, when activated together, stabilize the spine, and allow for postural stability, which is the muscle activity necessary to sit, stand, and move. The four sets of muscles surrounding the core are: 1) the diaphragm muscle from above, 2) the pelvic floor muscles from below, 3) the transverse abdominis (deepest of the four abdominals) at the front, and 4) the multifidus (deep back muscles) on the back. Together, they are the deep stabilizing system that forms the basis of our spine and posture stability.

When these muscles are activated together, they create intra-abdominal pressure. Think of a can of soda. The liquid pushes out against the can in all directions, making the thin aluminum tight and hard to squeeze, but when the fluid and the pressure are gone, the can easily crumples. In the body, this hydraulic pressure regulates the stability of the pelvis and lower back. The pressure reinforces the muscles that stabilize the spine, allowing you to maintain an upright, optimal posture from your pelvis to your neck. When everything is working correctly, you do this without even realizing it. But when there's a problem, you really feel it.

The problem most people have is not a lack of strength. A baby can properly stabilize their core as early as three months, allowing them to lift their arms and raise their head for the first time, all without ever having done any sit-ups or crunches. The most common problem comes in not activating the muscles properly. In this case, the core needs to be found and discovered just like you did in the first year of life. You need to feel it, be able to engage it, and control it.

A baby doesn't do core exercises to strengthen its core. Every position a baby holds and every move it tries to make is a core exercise. A baby naturally feels the stability that the deep stabilizing system creates and understands that this stability is necessary to move. Moving is ingrained in our nervous system from the earliest age. Thus, it becomes a positive feedback loop. The intra-abdominal pressure creates stability in the pelvis and back; that stability stabilizes the entire spine, establishing the basis for the muscles that move our head, arms, and legs. That's how a baby learns to move; the same principle applies as we age.

Over time, however, our posture and muscle imbalances can become more pronounced, and our ability to stabilize our spine can become less than ideal, causing pain and other problems. When that happens, strengthening your abs isn't the answer. To address the root causes, you must learn how to activate, engage, and control your stabilizing system.

Myth: Sit-Ups and Crunches Strengthen Your Core

We've all heard that sit-ups and crunches are the best way to strengthen your core. Not true. They may make your neck and back issues worse in some cases.

Sit-ups, curl-ups, and crunches are a mainstay of fitness programs. You will find them in personal training sessions, group exercise classes, Pilates, Yoga, at CrossFit gyms, online videos, and even the Presidential Youth Fitness Program they had us all doing in elementary school.

But you're not in elementary school anymore. As you age, sit-ups can be counterproductive for strengthening the core and may lead to or exacerbate chronic neck and back problems.

We all develop postural muscle imbalances over time. There are multiple reasons for this, but the simple answer is that different muscles serve specific purposes. Some muscles provide stability. These tend to be deeper, shorter muscles closer to our joints. Along with ligaments, they help protect our joints and spine by maintaining control around them, keeping static positions, and maintaining balance and posture in daily activities such as sitting or standing.

Other muscles are used primarily for movement. They tend to be superficial muscles (closer to the surface), longer, and further away from our joints. The contraction of these muscles creates the force that moves our limbs. For example, the quad muscles in the front of the thigh extend your lower leg and straighten your knee. The deltoid muscle outside your shoulder raises your arms against gravity. These muscles are dynamic and allow us to perform everyday actions such as walking, kicking a ball, and reaching for things.

A typical imbalance of our midsection occurs in the stabilizing muscles in our stomach and back. An overactive rectus abdominis (the

6-pack muscle) and overactive back paraspinals (the muscles that run up and down either side of the spine) can result from faulty posture, non-optimal breathing patterns, and poor deep spinal stability.

Sit-ups primarily train your rectus abdominis muscle, so you are contracting and strengthening an overly contracted and overactive muscle, to begin with. Many of my patients with chronic low back pain and abdominal pain instead have trigger points of their rectus abdominis. Treating these tight spots often eliminates their pain; no sit-ups are required.

I have also seen patients who caused neck symptoms by doing too many crunches or holding a sit-up for too long. This can happen when overcompensating with the superficial muscles in the front of the neck.

The underlying root cause of the problem is poor spinal and postural stability. However, it manifests as neck or back pain because of the overuse of the superficial muscles of the neck and back to compensate. These muscles were designed to make bigger movements, not provide stability.

Another scenario where sit-ups and curl-ups might be harmful or counterproductive for the back or neck is when dealing with a disc herniation. The crunching motion tends to exacerbate the disc herniation and produce pain, whether in the back or the neck.

That doesn't mean sit-ups, curl-ups, and crunches are never useful. When the deeper stabilizing system is engaged, we can safely use other muscles on top of that system to move in a balanced way that doesn't overload or strain our muscles. The best way is to learn how to engage your deeper core stability before and throughout the exercise so that we can move more safely and efficiently, with greater control and even better strength.

Myth: Your Core Is Strong Because You Do Core Exercises Regularly

Core exercises help strengthen your core, right? You can find an endless list of "core" exercises online or in any health or sports magazine. They are a part of any Pilates or Yoga class. You probably know the names: plank, side plank, bridge, flutter kicks, v-crunch, mountain climbers, bird dog, dead bug, superman, and so many more. The problem is not the exercise itself. All these exercises may very well be suitable for strengthening your core. The question is whether they are done correctly and within your current capability.

Remember that the core involves intra-abdominal pressure created by the four sets of muscles that make up the trunk. For that system to work, there must be an optimal relationship between the lower rib cage and the pelvis. They should be parallel to one another, with the lower rib cage stacked on top of the pelvis. This ensures that the diaphragm and pelvic floor will be optimally activated against each other.

Furthermore, the sound quality of core activation is necessary to benefit from the training without compensation. The quality is dictated by maintaining this proper relationship, maintaining pressure, elongating the spine while preserving optimal posture, and continuing steady breathing throughout the exercise without compensation or overloading other body parts.

The other problem is the difficulty. An exercise that is too difficult can do more harm than good. For example, the V-sit is an advanced core exercise. It involves lying on your back and bringing your straightened legs and chest up in unison so that your body assumes a V shape. This exercise takes quite a bit of core strength to maintain proper alignment, abdominal bracing, and steady breathing. For most people I see in the clinic, this exercise is too advanced. Some have said they tweaked their back or neck doing this exercise in Pilates or a group class at their gym.

It's essential to know that you are training your core stability at an appropriate level. Too easy won't maximize the benefit—too hard risks overloading other aspects of your body by compensating. If excess force is placed on your discs and joints because you couldn't maintain stability and alignment throughout the exercise, you could overload your spinal segments. If you compensate for weak stabilization by using muscles that aren't designed to stabilize, you can end up with muscle strains, tears, and painful trigger points. Trying the V-sit before you are ready, for instance, could injure the discs, joints, and muscles in your back and neck or, depending on the compensation, strain the muscles in your hips and shoulders.

Core exercises are great, but only when done correctly. The key is to have the body awareness and knowledge to maintain optimal postural alignment and core stability necessary for the given exercise. Then you can train within your limits without the risk of injury.

Myth: Pulling Your Belly Inward Engages the Core

Before introducing my patients to the core and spinal and postural stability concepts, I often ask them to demonstrate how they engage their core. Go ahead, try it yourself.

Most of the time, my patients will suck their bellies in. Did you do the same? When I ask them where they learned to do that, they will usually say something like, "my trainer told me to pull my stomach in" or "my Pilates instructor told me to pull my belly button up and in towards my spine," or that they read it in a fitness magazine or saw it online.

This is entirely INCORRECT. Pulling your belly button inward or sucking your stomach in does not engage your core. It does the opposite; it disengages the core and creates postural instability.

Why? First, it causes you to lift your chest and rib cage upwards. When the chest and rib cage are elevated towards your head, it limits the diaphragm's movement. This hurts the diaphragm's natural functions of respiration and stabilization. From a biomechanical standpoint, you can't engage your core optimally when your chest and rib cage are elevated because it takes the diaphragm out of the equation.

Second, pulling your belly in causes a contraction of your superficial abdominal muscles, which also limits the ability of the core to be engaged most optimally. It produces the same contraction that doing sit-ups and crunches does, but like those exercises, it doesn't engage the whole core.

A better way to think about engaging your core is to "pressurize" your stomach or "push out against your waistband." This cue will lower the rib cage, ensuring the diaphragm can play along. Now the diaphragm can be the stable roof of the core against the pelvic floor, while the deep abdominals form the front wall and the deep back muscles form the back wall. This coactivation creates the intra-abdominal pressure that stabilizes the spine and forms the basis of our postural stability. The martial arts have figured this out, which is why they commonly teach students to exhale or yell through punches and kicks. Forceful exhalation depresses the diaphragm downward, which helps to engage the core, thus giving more efficiency and power to the punch or kick.

Try this quick demonstration for yourself. Put one hand on your chest and one hand on your belly. Now suck your stomach in or pull your belly button toward your spine. Notice what happens to the belly hand and your chest hand. The belly hand is drawn inward toward your body, and the chest hand is drawn upward. Maintain this position by pulling your stomach in and now punch each arm in front of you several times. Pay attention to your body and posture. How does it feel?

Go back to the starting position with one hand on your chest and one on your belly. This time, forcibly exhale by saying "shhh" or blowing air out quickly. You should feel your abdominal wall pushing out against you with your belly hand and your chest depressing downward toward your feet. Next, maintain that pressurized feeling as you punch your arms out again. How do your body and posture feel now? Which feels better, more efficient, more stable, and stronger?

Myth: Correct Your Posture by Lifting Your Chest and Squeezing Your Shoulders Back

Throughout childhood, we have all been told "sit up straight" and "don't slouch." In adulthood, good posture has become increasingly important in maintaining our well-being and optimal health, especially when our society has shown trends of increased time spent watching television, sitting in front of computers, working sedentary desk jobs, and commuting long hours. But do those childhood instructions still apply?

To answer that, we need to know more about posture's role in our optimal health and core stability.

Poor posture over the long term has been associated with numerous painful conditions relating to the function of muscles, joints, ligaments, nerves, connective tissue, circulation, respiration, and digestion. Commonly diagnosed conditions associated with poor posture include temporomandibular joint dysfunction, headaches, neck pain, shoulder pain, repetitive strain injuries, mid and low back pain, thoracic outlet syndrome, and myofascial pain syndrome. In addition, poor sitting posture may adversely affect activities of daily living and decrease overall energy levels at work and home.

The concept of a single, static, ideal posture is misleading. It doesn't consider that people have a genetic predisposition towards a specific spinal alignment or that a person needs multiple positions to accomplish tasks in varying situations. Other factors that influence our postures include the environment surrounding us, our habits, and our attitudes at a certain point in time. So, there is no one perfect posture. Posture is dynamic. Our bodies constantly react to and work against gravity and other stresses to maintain a functional balance.

Good sitting posture indeed maintains the normal curvatures of the lumbar (lower back), thoracic (mid-back), and cervical (neck) spine, allowing the body and head to be upright with minimal muscular effort. However, a prolonged, static sitting position will eventually lead to feelings of stiffness, soreness, achiness, and pain as body tissues become overloaded.

The most common improper sitting posture is slouching, characterized by a rounded lower back, humped upper back, rounded shoulders, and a forward head position. The resulting alignment can lead to muscle imbalances, connective tissue restrictions, altered shoulder and spinal joint mechanics, increased vertebral disc compression, and narrowing of the space in which arteries and nerves pass. Poor posture makes you vulnerable to injury and hinders healing and adequate resolution of associated painful conditions.

So, should we all be following our childhood advice? If I ask a patient to show me how to correct their posture in a sitting and standing position, they always do the same thing: pull their chest up and bring their shoulders back, just as they were told as a child. However, this cue is not the best and can lead to more neck and back dysfunction.

At first glance, it may look like this chest-up-shoulders-back correction quickly straightens the posture, but this is misleading. The main problem is that it compromises the relationship between the lower rib cage and pelvis. It puts the pelvis in a forward tilted position and elevates the lower rib cage. This position of the pelvis and rib cage increases tension and activity in the muscles of the lower back and between the shoulder blades, overloads the lower spine, compromises the ability to breathe fully, and inhibits the ability to engage the core.

Try it for yourself. Sit at the edge of a chair. Lift your chest and bring your shoulder blades back. Hold this position for 10 seconds and try to take full breaths. What do you feel? Do you notice any tension in your lower back, shallow breathing, or even back pain? You are not alone. This is not an optimal posture. Before you worry about your chest, shoulders, and head position, you must first align your pelvis and lower rib cage. Otherwise, you may be doing more harm than good.

Myth: Stretching Out Tight Muscles Is the Best Way to Address Muscle Imbalances

The efficient and coordinated use of the body requires many different muscles working together. When one group of muscles is longer or stronger than another opposing group, whether in the same limb or on the opposite side of the body, things can start to break down. This is called a muscle imbalance.

For example, you may have experienced tight hamstrings. The hamstrings, when contracted, flex the knee. If they are too tight, they may limit the range of motion, preventing you from straightening the knee. Another typical example is an overly tight and dominant outer quad muscle versus a weak and inhibited inner quad muscle that causes the kneecap to move to the outside when the quad contracts. This movement can contribute to the dysfunction of the joints in your kneecap.

Muscles can become imbalanced due to either adaptation or dysfunction. An adaptive or functional imbalance is an imbalance that results from poor posture or participation in habitual sport, work, and lifestyle activities. If you sit at a desk in the same way for 20-30 years, your body will naturally adapt to that position, whether it is a proper position or not.

Dysfunctional imbalances are changes that result from trauma, pain, or surgery. A person who suffers pain from an injury may compensate and move in an altered way to avoid pain, even long after the pain has subsided. For example, if you have pain in your big toe, you will probably alter how you walk to avoid moving the toe as much as possible. This change can then affect all the parts of your body involved in walking.

In most muscle or postural imbalances, some muscles are prone to getting tight and shortened, while others are prone to be inhibited and weak. If we look at the first problem (tight and shortened muscles), it makes sense to work on the flexibility of these muscles through stretching exercises. Think of those pesky tight muscles you are aware of in your own body; you may have caught yourself trying to stretch them to relieve the tension or discomfort.

Muscle flexibility is essential but stretching alone is not enough to lengthen or decrease the tone of a muscle. Other ways to reduce tension in an overly tight muscle include foam rolling, self-massage with a small ball, and releasing trigger points. These aspects of soft tissue mobilization are important to allow for greater flexibility and length in a shortened muscle.

However, stretching out tight muscles only fixes one part of the problem. Activating or strengthening inhibited and weak muscles are essential too. For example, weak gluteal muscles may adversely affect your back, hip, or knee pain. Strengthening these butt muscles helps reduce the imbalance in the hip or lower spine, which affects how you walk, from your legs to your knees to your feet. Anyone who has ever worked with a personal trainer or physical therapist knows the importance of strengthening underdeveloped muscles with targeted exercises and the enormous difference it can make.

Myth: Chin Tucks and Back Rows Will Fix Your Faulty Posture

Just because exercises can help activate or strengthen weak muscles doesn't mean that all exercises are equally good or even accomplish what you might think they do. Some may be hurting you. To explain, let's look at two common postural exercises: chin tucks and resisted back rows.

A chin tuck involves tucking in your chin as if you were nodding yes. It can be done lying down, sitting, or standing and is often given to people to improve their forward head posture. Usually, the exercise is meant to be held for 10 seconds or longer to improve the activation and endurance of the deep neck flexors found along the front side of your spine at your neck.

The resisted back row has you sitting or standing with your arms straight out, holding a resistance band, squeezing your shoulders together and pulling your elbows back to the side of your body like rowing a boat. Usually, the movement is repeated for several sets but can also be held to work on endurance. This exercise is often intended to improve a forward-rounded shoulder position.

On the surface, it may seem logical that these two exercises would address poor posture. However, they don't train your body to maintain good posture naturally because they fail to account for how we all learned to sit, stand, walk, and move from our earliest days as infants until now.

We should stop training with isolated movements and exercises that do not consider what is necessary for our body to stabilize and upright itself against gravity. Otherwise, we are building strength on top of a weak foundation, resulting in more compensation, more non-optimal patterns of movement, more overloading of tissue, more dysfunction, and more pain. This is the secret to finding the root cause of many chronic neck and back issues.

The way to fix our posture is to train our stability system and coordinated motor control, just like when we were babies. We eventually progress to a chin tuck or squeeze our shoulder blades together, but only once we have corrected our deeper stabilizing system. This is how we stop having surface-level problems and start getting stronger from the inside out.

Truth: You Develop Your Posture as a Baby, and You Still Can Improve It as You Age

In the first year of life, we develop our deep spinal stability system, which creates the postural stability necessary to lift our head, move our limbs, sit, stand, and walk. This early development process is an absolute wonder, but it is something that most of us take for granted.

Does a baby do sit-ups to strengthen their core? Does a baby do sets of chin tucks to strengthen their deep neck flexors? Does a baby do resisted rows to strengthen the back muscles? Do you have to remind them to keep their chest up and shoulders back or to sit up straight? Of course not. Although, it would be funny to see them try.

So how did we learn how to create the spinal and postural stability necessary to sit upright against gravity and stand in a balanced way? Around the third month, a baby's central nervous system becomes more developed and purposeful. The baby is curious and is ingrained to begin moving. They hear, see, and sense the world around them and are eager to explore. They begin to feel and be aware of the ability to create abdominal pressure coordinated with their breath. This intra-abdominal pressure starts a cascade of coordinated activation of the deep spine flexors and extensors. The resultant muscle activity creates an elongation of the spine up the neck to the base of the head. This is the initial activation and stability the baby needs to make small movements, lifting the head, arms, and legs.

The ability to do it is not great initially, but they slowly progress to more significant movements for extended periods. This creates enough stability to turn on to their side and then to their stomach. Then they learn how to stabilize, starting with intra-abdominal pressure, moving their limbs and supporting themselves with their arms, eventually supporting with their elbows and being able to lift their head and look around and see the world in a whole new way.

The baby learns to create stability through one arm (resting on the elbow and shoulder) to reach for something with the other arm. Same for the legs. They may even begin to crawl on their stomach. They wish to explore and are determined to move. As they age, the baby continues to find new ways to stabilize and move in different positions, and their endurance improves over time.

Eventually, the baby can side-sit propped on a hand and a hip. Then they learn to sit, testing stability in that position by reaching for things. They fail and learn, fail, and learn, constantly improving their stability and endurance to hold positions for longer and longer periods.

Next, they begin crawling, supporting their body on arms and legs. From there, they advance their mobility to half-kneeling, to squatting, to standing, assisted at first by the furniture or the wall, until finally, they can do it independently.

Over the course of nine to twelve months, the baby has completely trained their motor control from nothing, starting helplessly on their back to running around the table like a tiny Tasmanian devil. It all began with coordinating their breath and deeper stability when they were three months old. We can take advantage of the same basic principles to retrain our bodies the way we first learned, no matter our age.

CHAPTER 2

Mistakes People Make in Addressing Chronic Neck & Back Pain

"When solving problems, dig at the roots instead of just hacking at the leaves."

Anthony J. D'Angelo

Treating the Symptoms and Not Addressing the Underlying Root Cause

Look at the remedies available to treat spine pain—cold and heating pads, pain-relieving creams and ointments, electrical stimulation devices, braces, inversion traction tables, over-the-counter pain medicines, prescription medicines, steroid injections, and so on. Although these methods may relieve the pain in the short term, they don't address the root cause of the pain.

There is nothing wrong with treating the pain–it's important and valuable–but it won't necessarily result in long-term relief or the prevention of future recurrent problems. Treating the pain may dampen or temporarily extinguish the fire, but it won't address what ignited it.

Back pain treated by orthopedists, physical therapists, and chiropractors is often due to a displaced disc herniation. A disc herniation is a weakening or tear in the outer layers of a spinal disc, which causes the inner part of the disc to displace backward or to the side, potentially compressing or irritating existing nerve roots from the spine. The condition is mainly seen in people aged 20 to 50.

The pain usually starts in the back and then radiates down to the front, side, or back of the leg. Sometimes the pain is just in the leg and not the back. It may happen over time or suddenly, as when bending over to pick up an object. Once it happens, it often comes back again and again. Bending, twisting, sitting, prolonged positions, and coughing or sneezing cause excessive pain, which may be worse in the morning, and it may be challenging to stand up after sitting for a while. While standing, it can be difficult to stand straight, causing a shift to one side. Rest or lying down may improve it somewhat.

A person with this type of back pain usually sees their primary care doctor or an orthopedist first. The doctor will often give medication such as muscle relaxers or pain-relieving, anti-inflammatory meds in addition to general advice. For an ongoing problem, an X-ray or an MRI is usually taken. If the pain is intense enough, they may refer them to a pain management specialist to receive a steroid injection.

After all that, the doctor may, but does not always, send them to a physical therapist. By the time a patient receives any physical therapy, months may have passed from when they were injured. Every intervention this person received in the meantime was aimed at treating the symptoms, from the general advice to the medications to the steroid injection. Disc herniation causes nerve compression or nerve sensitivity due to inflammation, producing pain. So, to the extent that the irritated nerve is causing the person's pain, all these meds, oral steroids, and injections might give some relief.

But what's causing the nerve to be irritated? The disc herniation. But we are still not at the root of the problem. What's causing the disc herniation? The answer is likely to be excessive load forces acting on the spine, which causes the outer layers of the disc to get weak and, eventually, herniated. No amount of meds will do anything to correct that or keep it from recurring.

The lack of spinal stability explains the numerous past episodes. It's often not the acute event itself. Bending over to pick up a pencil should not lead to a disc herniation. Instead, the straw that broke the camel's back happened because spinal instability caused excessive spine compression gradually over time. The accumulation of minor episodes leads to an inevitable major episode with debilitating pain and functional disability.

Many small factors can cause this harmful stress on the spine, and only by working to address those factors can permanent relief be achieved. Some of those factors may be easy to change (such as proper posture and desk ergonomics), other factors may be hard to change (such as excessive body weight), and some aspects are unable to change (such as genetic predisposition). However, one thing that everyone can improve upon is the capacity of the deep spinal and postural stability system. Improving your core stability pushes back against your spine, giving it support and allowing it to elongate, fighting against the compression.

The solution to the underlying issue is stabilizing the spine against load forces from the inside out. You must train your core stability system to act appropriately when the circumstances call for it. This is the long-term fix for many chronic neck and back sufferers, a way to get mobility and freedom back without fear of recurring episodes and an endless stream of medications and injections.

Too Much Reliance on Medical Professionals, Tests, and Imaging

Low back pain is common worldwide and affects most people, of all ages and income classes, at some point in their life. It is estimated that 80% of people will suffer a disabling episode of back pain during their lifetime. One episode of disabling back pain doesn't mean that you will always have back pain from that point on, but approximately 5% to 10% of cases will develop into chronic low back pain.[1] In fact, low back pain is now the leading cause of disability globally.[2]

---

[1] (MEUCCI, R. D., FASSA, A. G., & FARIA, N. M. (2015). PREVALENCE OF CHRONIC LOW BACK PAIN: SYSTEMATIC REVIEW. REVISTA DE SAUDE PUBLICA, 49, 1. https://doi.org/10.1590/S0034-8910.2015049005874)

[2] (HARTVIGSEN, J., HANCOCK, M. J., KONGSTED, A., LOUW, Q., FERREIRA, M. L., GENEVAY, S., HOY, D., KARPPINEN, J., PRANSKY, G., SIEPER, J., SMEETS, R. J., UNDERWOOD, M., & LANCET LOW BACK PAIN SERIES WORKING GROUP (2018). WHAT LOW BACK PAIN IS AND WHY WE NEED TO PAY ATTENTION. LANCET (LONDON, ENGLAND), 391(10137), 2356–2367. https://doi.org/10.1016/S0140-6736(18)30480-X)

Similar statistics are accurate with chronic neck pain. According to the Mayo Clinic, "neck pain is the fourth leading cause of disability, with an annual prevalence exceeding 30%. Most episodes of acute neck pain will resolve with or without treatment, but nearly 50% of individuals will continue to experience some degree of pain or frequent occurrences."[3]

These numbers are staggering, and the cost to our society is enormous. Anyone dealing with chronic neck or lower back pain knows the consequences affect almost every aspect of their life, from work to recreation to family to personal and mental wellbeing.

Chronic neck and back pain are the most common problems I've treated in my physical therapy career over the past 23 years. Every time I take someone's history and hear their story, I think about the underlying factors that have led to this epidemic of disability. The individual reasons for pain vary, but I have noticed a common thread in how their stories progress from a painful episode to a chronic disability. In nearly every case, they received inappropriate or inadequate interventions from the first line of medical providers, whether an emergency room physician, primary care physician, orthopedic physician, physical therapist, or chiropractor.

In the US, it is not uncommon for someone with a neck or back issue to see a doctor first, usually their primary care physician, unless it's a severe episode, in which case they may see an emergency room

---

[3] (COHEN S. P. (2015), EPIDEMIOLOGY, DIAGNOSIS, AND TREATMENT OF NECK PAIN. MAYO CLINIC PROCEEDINGS, 90(2), 284–299. https://doi.org/10.1016/j.mayocp.2014.09.008)

physician. Most will go to a doctor first if you ask someone what they would do for a neck or back problem. However, these medical professionals are not truly equipped to evaluate a neck or lower back condition.

That might sound judgmental and opinionated, but it's true. Primary care or an ER physician must deal with all sorts of general health problems, so it is not a surprise they aren't experts at any given specialty, particularly one as complex as this. You wouldn't expect a primary care physician to be the top expert on a brain tumor, so why would you expect them to be the only person needed to treat your back pain?

This is not the case in other countries, including the Netherlands, where I received some of my physical therapy education. A person with a musculoskeletal problem, such as neck or back pain, sees a physical therapist first because they are specifically trained to examine these types of spinal conditions.

When I ask new patients with neck and back pain what happened at their primary care doctor or emergency room visit, I hear a familiar story. A thorough history wasn't taken (often less than 10 minutes), followed by general advice to rest and give it time, along with pain medications. Take this, give it time, and you'll be fine.

The worst part, only 7% of those who go to a primary care physician with low back pain are referred for physical therapy.[4]

---

[4] Fritz, J. M., Childs, J. D., Wainner, R. S., & Flynn, T. W. (2012). Primary care referral of patients with low back pain to physical therapy: impact on

Many physicians are trained to recognize red flags that might indicate severe pathologies, such as a fracture or cancer. In most cases, however, acute back pain is not due to serious pathology. Instead, it's neuromusculoskeletal in nature. Thus, the numbers should be reversed. 93% should be referred to physical therapy first. Physical therapy costs less, results in better clinical outcomes, and decreases subsequent use of prescription medication, MRI scans, and injections.[5]

Another problem that can arise at the doctor's office involves the introduction of imaging. After a month or two of persistent pain, the patient returns to the doctor. The general advice and medication have failed to solve the problem; and the next step is often to order an X-ray or MRI to see exactly what is happening.

However, you usually don't need an X-ray or an MRI to confirm an arthritic spine, disc herniation, or compressed and irritated spinal nerve. Any good clinician can determine that from a good history and physical examination. X-rays and MRIs should be saved for the cases that don't respond to conservative treatment or those showing signs of neurological compromise. Unnecessary scans only increase patient anxiety and pave the way for further medical and surgical interventions that may not be needed.

FUTURE HEALTH CARE UTILIZATION AND COSTS. SPINE, 37(25), 2114–2121. https://doi.org/10.1097/BRS.0b013e31825d32f5)

[5] (FRITZ, J. M., CLELAND, J. A., SPECKMAN, M., BRENNAN, G. P., & HUNTER, S. J. (2008). PHYSICAL THERAPY FOR ACUTE LOW BACK PAIN: ASSOCIATIONS WITH SUBSEQUENT HEALTHCARE COSTS. SPINE, 33(16), 1800–1805. https://doi.org/10.1097/BRS.0b013e31817bd853)

But isn't it harmless to run a scan, just in case, to see what is going on? No. The harm comes in the form of unnecessary and problematic interventions. Most of the time, a scan is going to find something. Depending on your age, it will discover compressed degenerative spines, herniated discs, or nerves that do not have much space. By 30, most people show some early signs of degenerative changes in the neck and lower back. But that doesn't mean everyone needs surgery when they turn 30.

Also, a scan can't tell you exactly what's wrong with your spine. It gives you a snapshot of your spine in the position when you get the image taken. An MRI of your spine while lying on your back gives little indication of how your spine functions in a weight-bearing position such as sitting, standing, or walking. It provides a minimal representation of what's happening with functional activities such as bending, twisting, and moving.

So many poor decisions have been made in the history of people's chronic neck and back problems based on inadequate early interventions and imaging results. I hear about them in my clinic all the time, people who were not even taken through a physical examination, who then got a steroid injection or surgery that did not correlate with their actual problem. By the time they come to me, they are worse off than when they started because they never addressed the underlying causes of their pain.

We have it backward. We put doctors, medication, and invasive procedures before conservative, therapeutic measures. This inversion is a significant factor in our society's prevalence and the propensity for chronic spine problems. But it's completely avoidable. We need a dramatic shift away from the reliance on imaging and toward an emphasis on thorough evaluations and appropriate referrals to clinicians who can conservatively address the underlying problems. I have hundreds of patients who can testify to the results.

Thinking That Surgery Will Fix Chronic Neck and Back Pain

No one wants to have surgery, but if it's the only option left, at least you know it will solve the problem, right? It's a common belief that spinal surgery, as a last resort, will always work, especially for debilitating chronic low back pain. Unfortunately, this isn't true.

There is a time and place for spinal surgery. Spine surgeons are excellent at what they do and have helped countless people live better lives. But over the past few decades, researchers have discovered some disturbing trends regarding the prevalence and effectiveness of spinal surgical procedures.

The number of spinal fusion surgical procedures rose 62% between 2004 and 2015 in the United States. Spinal fusion may be appropriate for spinal deformity and structural spinal instability. Still, its efficacy for disc degeneration, herniation, and spinal stenosis has not been established, yet this group accounted for 42% of total elective lumbar fusions in 2015.[6]

---

[6] Martin, B. I., Mirza, S. K., Spina, N., Spiker, W. R., Lawrence, B., & Brodke, D. S. (2019). Trends in Lumbar Fusion Procedure Rates and Associated Hospital

Anatomical deformities of the spine are typically due to underlying pathology. Scoliosis is a perfect example. Spinal instability describes structural instability among the vertebrae, such as slippage of one vertebra over another, which can impinge on nerves or even the spinal cord. The medical diagnosis for this is spondylolisthesis. It can be caused by genetics, a significant trauma such as a car accident, or repeated stressful loads over time, as in a young athlete.

A spinal fusion may be required for such problems, as spinal deformities can adversely affect growth development and the function of major organs. Still, it should not be taken lightly. Not every person with scoliosis needs a spinal fusion. The same is true for spinal instabilities. Spinal fusions may be recommended for specific spinal issues, especially if they are causing progressive neurological compromise when the risk of not doing the procedure is irreversible nerve damage and more significant disability.

Non-instability neck and back problems are related to the spine's structures, including the disc, the joints, and the nerves. Common diagnoses include disc herniations, degenerative disc disease, spondylosis (spinal joint arthritis), and spinal stenosis.

Disc herniations are spinal conditions where the outer layers of the disc weaken and tear, causing a part of the disc to herniate, possibly irritating or compressing nerves. Disc and joint degeneration,

---

Costs for Degenerative Spinal Diseases in the United States, 2004 to 2015. *Spine*, 44(5), 369–376. https://doi.org/10.1097/BRS.0000000000002822

commonly known as degenerative disc disease or spinal spondylosis, is arthritis of the spine. This wear and tear on the spine's discs and joints that happen over time can also irritate and compress nerves coming out of the spine and eventually lead to spinal stenosis, which is the narrowing of spaces within the spine. It commonly occurs where the spinal cord runs (central spinal stenosis) or where the spinal nerve roots exit (lateral spinal stenosis). These problems can be due to several factors and are routinely addressed conservatively.

There are times, however, when a spinal surgery procedure could be necessary when conservative measures haven't worked or when a neurological compromise is progressive in nature and leads toward a loss of function. The procedure is called spinal discectomies or spinal laminectomies, where part of the disc and bone is removed to alleviate pressure or create space around the nerve. Rarely, and only for severe cases, would a spinal fusion be necessary for these types of conditions. Yet nearly half (42%) of spinal fusion procedures were performed for these non-instability types of spinal problems.[7]

Other conditions where spinal procedures are all too common are chronic neck pain, chronic back pain, or chronic pain syndrome. This is neck or back pain that has caused persistently high levels of pain and disability, has affected the person's psychological state but has not responded to treatment. Often, there is no clear indication of a specific structural problem, as with the cases above. In this case, it is doubtful

---

[7] Martin, B. I., Mirza, S. K., Spina, N., Spiker, W. R., Lawrence, B., & Brodke, D. S. (2019). Trends in Lumbar Fusion Procedure Rates and Associated Hospital Costs for Degenerative Spinal Diseases in the United States, 2004 to 2015. *Spine, 44*(5), 369–376. https://doi.org/10.1097/BRS.0000000000002822

that a spinal procedure, especially a spinal fusion procedure, will help. They will generally be much better off learning to address and manage their pain through less invasive and costly means. Just because someone has been suffering from spine pain for a long time doesn't mean that surgery will solve all their problems.

Surgery is designed to correct specific structural problems, but chronic pain is complex. Simply removing something from your spine or fusing your vertebrae will not necessarily make all the various factors that lead to pain disappear. In fact, if the underlying cause of the problem is not addressed, surgery could make things worse, leading to a spiral of more pain, more problems, and more surgeries. For example, it is not uncommon for the spinal fusion of two vertebrae to lead to the degeneration of the spinal segments above or below the fusion. Over time, the pain will return, and more fusions will be needed if the root causes are not corrected.

If you only take measures to remove or alter the structural problem, you will not address the underlying issues that caused the structure to become compromised. The way to get long-lasting relief is first to address the functional factors that cause stress, strain, and compression of the spinal structures. Only once that is done can surgery be successfully used to correct structural problems, and only when necessary for a specific diagnosis.

Not Understanding the Signs of Spinal and Postural Instability

Spinal instability falls into two basic categories: structural and clinical. Structural spine instability is when the spine structure is compromised to the extent of causing significant adverse alignment and neurological implications that usually require a surgical fix. Clinical spinal instability is when the spine structure is compromised to the extent that although it may be causing symptoms or loss of function, it does not yet have significant, irreversible problems. Physicians or surgeons treat structural cases, while physical therapists or chiropractors treat clinical cases.

The problem is that when someone has the symptoms of neck or back instability, they usually see a doctor, orthopedist, or spine surgeon first. Since they primarily treat structural instabilities, this diagnosis will be at the front of their mind. They will often order an X-ray or MRI to detect any structural defects. But what happens when the imaging studies don't show significant instability? They are not experienced in handling this type of a patient, so they may miss the signs of clinical spinal instability and may not know how to treat it outside their standard procedures.

Unfortunately, most spinal instabilities fall into this clinical category, so most people don't get adequate treatment or advice from their healthcare professionals. Instead, they are submitted to useless scans or told there is nothing they can do but rest and wait for it to get worse.

But there are plenty of ways to treat clinical instability if you recognize the signs and get the right help.

Here are some examples of the signs and symptoms of clinical spinal instability, whether in the neck or back:

- Chronic pain in the neck and back
- Repeated episodes of neck or back pain
- The feeling your neck or back is going to give out
- The feeling your neck or back locks or gets stuck during specific movements
- Clicking, popping, crunching, crackling sounds in the joints of your neck or back
- Neck or back pain when changing positions (rolling out of bed, getting up out of a chair, etc.)
- Worsening neck or back pain in prolonged or static positions
- The need to pop or crack your neck or back
- Frequent neck or back muscle tension or spasms

Maybe these sound familiar. Clinical spinal and postural instability is prevalent and the underlying cause of many people's chronic neck and back problems. It may or may not show up on imaging, and there is no bloodwork to diagnose it, but there are physical tests that a clinician can perform to add more certainty to these signs.

If these signs and symptoms were more routinely and quickly recognized by first-line healthcare professionals and the appropriate referral was made to a physical therapist, chiropractor, or personal trainer who has training and expertise in addressing spinal and postural instability, we would negate much of the push for medications, injections, and surgical interventions that do not address the problem. The sooner it's recognized and managed, the lesser the chance of the situation becoming a chronic issue that often leads to pain, disability, and the loss of joy that comes from being afflicted by pain and physical limitations.

Not Recognizing the Significant Role of Muscle Imbalances

Nobody gets through life without developing muscle imbalances. If you practice yoga or stretch regularly, you may have noticed differences between a muscle on one side of your body and the same muscle on the other side. I often hear people say they have tight hamstrings or tight hip flexors. Some people will notice the differences in their dominant arm and shoulder compared to their non-dominant arm and shoulder. If you are living, you are changing, and your body is adapting to various influences that affect different body parts to various degrees, causing one part to grow stronger and another weaker, one part being tight and another loose. Often, these changes happen so gradually that we don't notice them until years later.

Many influences on our postural and muscle imbalances exist. They may be genetics, early childhood physical development, the environment, or painful traumas. Some people are genetically predisposed to scoliosis (a curvature of the spine), overly rounded mid-back (thoracic kyphosis), or internally rotated hips. These structural influences will affect how your muscles function around them, sometimes leading to imbalances.

Development during the first stages of life can also influence future muscle imbalances. How you first learn to move can also set you up for compensatory movement patterns that influence your behavior and structure for your whole life. So can your daily environment. Sitting behind a desk for years can contribute to muscle imbalances, as can the position you sleep in, the sports you play, and the repetitive work you do.

Finally, painful traumas can significantly influence muscle imbalances, including minor injuries, significant traumas (emotional or physical), and surgeries. Our nervous system aims to avoid pain, so any painful experience will cause us to compensate somehow. A sore toe affects how you walk, just as a kink in your neck affects how you move your head. Even after the noticeable pain is gone, the faulty movement patterns can remain, causing muscle imbalances over time.

Muscle imbalances are a problem because they affect how you maintain your static and dynamic postures. The spine varies between stiff areas and more mobile areas, and these mobile areas, where the spine hinges or curves, are particularly susceptible to excess stress, movement, and strain. Think of the angle between the head and the upper neck, the lower neck and the upper back, the lower mid-back and the upper lower back, and the lower back and the tailbone. If you do not have optimal posture, these areas can begin to move too much and into wrong positions, creating further strain and stress. This is also true for your extremity joints. Muscle imbalances around a hip, for example, can contribute to excessive stress, compression, and strain in the hip joint, eventually leading to cartilage breakdown and arthritis.

Muscle imbalances can also alter your movement mechanics. When you add movement to the excessive stress and strain already occurring, the compression and excess load placed on already weak or damaged joints further their breakdown over time. And any imbalances between tight muscles and those that are inhibited or weak change the way the joints move, not in a positive way. The suboptimal movement patterns then put new stresses on your tissues and joints.

The shoulder is a perfect example of where this can occur. Muscle imbalances around the shoulder girdle often keep the shoulder in a forward position rather than a neutral one. When you raise that arm overhead, the ball in the socket of the glenohumeral joint doesn't move as smoothly or efficiently, which can cause a lack of space for your rotator cuff tendons to move. This is called shoulder impingement syndrome, a prevalent condition. This microtrauma over time contributes to the breakdown of the rotator cuff tendons and stress in the shoulder joint, leading to partial rotator cuff tears and joint cartilage breakdown that most of us are walking around with but wouldn't know about without an X-ray or MRI.

Muscle imbalances also overload and overburden muscles, causing even more tight and painful muscles. Some muscles are prone to get shortened and tight, while others are prone to lengthen and weaken.

Both these muscles can develop a trigger point, an exquisitely tender area in a muscle that causes generalized pain and transfers to other body parts when overstimulated. Not only can trigger points cause pain, but they also contribute to decreased flexibility, coordination, strength, and other dysfunctions. For this reason, dry needling, which is highly effective at releasing trigger points, has become an increasingly more common method of treating musculoskeletal pain and dysfunction.

In my experience, the most common muscle dysfunction of the neck is found in the overly tight and shortened upper trapezius and levator scapulae muscles. These two muscles attach from your shoulder blade to your neck and are often involved in chronic neck problems. They tend to be overworked, trying to compensate for lack of spinal and postural stability.

Another muscle group that tends to get tight is the pectoralis muscles in your chest and infraspinatus shoulder rotator cuff muscles. Tight pecs pull the shoulder girdle forward, which causes the infraspinatus to be lengthened and weak. Both are overburdened due to the imbalance of the shoulder girdle and are prone to being a source of pain and dysfunction.

Muscle imbalances can also limit the ability to breathe and stabilize the spine optimally. Overly tight superficial back and hip flexor muscles contribute to a pelvis that is rotated forward and a lower rib cage that is elevated. That imbalance and the resultant misalignment change the position of the diaphragm muscle at the bottom of the rib cage. With a high lower rib cage, the diaphragm is hindered in its primary function of descending into the abdomen when taking a breath. The result is a shallow breath, more in the chest than in the stomach, the exact reverse of what it should be. The imbalance also adversely affects the diaphragm in its second most important job of helping create intra-abdominal pressure. Both functional limitations significantly impact your ability to stabilize your spine, which is at the core of many people's chronic neck and back pain.

In summary, muscle and postural imbalances affect all of us and inhibit our body's ability to breathe, stabilize, and move at its best. This contributes to excessive loads and stress on our spine and joints, alters how our joints move, and overloads our muscles, causing painful trigger points. Over time, neuromusculoskeletal pain and dysfunction develop. Despite being one of the most straightforward explanations for our musculoskeletal problems, muscle imbalances are widely underappreciated and misunderstood amongst both the public and healthcare professionals. Addressing these imbalances through activities such as yoga, massage, and regular exercises to increase our core stability awareness, strength, and stamina, would go a long way toward eliminating the widespread musculoskeletal problems in our society.

Expecting a Quick Fix

We would all love to have a quick fix. It would be great to take a pill, get an injection, even have surgery, and have the pain go away forever. However, like most things in life, making a meaningful change takes time. Quick fixes are always temporary because they don't lead to a correction in the behavior or underlying condition that caused the problem in the first place. Lasting improvement requires a much deeper correction.

This is true of many health problems. Medication may be a quick fix if you develop high blood pressure, or your cholesterol numbers are getting too high. The pills will certainly lower your blood pressure or improve your cholesterol numbers. But is this addressing the problem, or will it return as soon as the medication stops? The real problem is likely to be weight and diet issues, lack of exercise, high stress levels, psychological anger or anxiety issues, etc. The medicine does nothing to address these core issues and may prevent you from ever addressing them by shielding you from the real consequences.

Most of us are blind to these root problems in various aspects of our health. Even if we realize the problem, we fail to address it because we think it will be too hard to fix or are afraid to give up the comfort we have created for ourselves. It is easier to carry on with our established habits, healthy or not, and to blame the resulting problems on our genes, parents, society, or whatever else. We opt for the pill because it's easier. It doesn't require anything of us.

The influence of genetics, upbringing, culture, environment, etc., may be real, but they are rarely in our control, which is why they make such a great excuse. On the other hand, we have control over what we put in our bodies, how much we move, our sleep quality, our stress, and how we deal with our emotional states. There are times when medication or other quick fixes are necessary to get through a difficult or painful time and avoid more significant damage. In those cases, it is good that we have them. However, we must recognize the risks and not let the allure of the quick fix or temporary relief keep us from addressing the underlying causes.

The quick fixes for acute neck and back are plentiful. There is no shortage of treatments and therapies that will offer relief, including pain-relieving creams and ointments, over-the-counter medications, prescription medications, electrical stimulation devices (TENS unit), cortisone injections, lidocaine injections, prolotherapy, plasma rich platelet (PRP) injections, supplements, braces, etc. However, the nature of any chronic condition is that it develops and occurs over time. No single medication or therapy can undo years of stress and dysfunction in a single treatment. They give immediate help to the pain of the moment but don't remove the root causes that will inevitably make the pain return.

Take the case of a person suffering from recurrent tension-type headaches. Physical examination reveals tight, painful neck muscles with active trigger points that refer pain in the head and reproduce the headache. Manual therapy and dry needling of the involved neck muscles will relieve the headache pain more often than not. This should not be discounted. It may seem like a minor miracle for someone who has suffered headaches that no one has been able to diagnose or treat. But the treatment can't end there. What caused the trigger point to be active and refer pain in the head? That answer may be poor posture, poor underlying spinal stability, recent stress, previous car accidents or trauma history, sedentary desk job, or a combination of these things. Tackling these issues is the only way to ensure the headaches don't keep returning after each successful treatment.

Or consider a person suffering from chronic neck and back pain who has received chiropractic spinal manipulation for years. They can describe how the manipulation relieves neck and back pain, but it's often short-lived, and they will say that they need to return regularly to keep it in check. It is fantastic that spinal manipulation provides relief from the pain, but is this solving the root cause of the problem? The lack of spinal mobility or spinal misalignment may cause immediate pain, but then what is causing the spine to get constantly stuck, misaligned, or stiff? That answer will bring you closer to the root of the problem. A lack of underlying spinal and postural stability is at the heart of spinal misalignments, hypermobility, and hypomobility. Long-term relief will come from treating these primary causes, not the secondary symptoms.

The common problem is getting tricked into thinking the problem is solved without ever searching deeper. The pain goes away, and we believe the problem is fixed. I see this play out in my practice every day. I will relieve a client's neck and back pain within a few sessions and get them back to moving and functioning better. Great! That's my goal. But when they feel better, they stop coming in for therapy.

Very often, they will come back three months later, maybe six months later, or one year later, or even three years later, and they will tell me their back went out again, worse than ever, or their neck locked up again after a bad night's sleep. They usually want more dry needling or manual therapy sessions that helped them the last time. I tell them I am happy to give them some instant relief, but I also say we must spend more time and energy managing the underlying causes, or they will return to my office again and again.

If you've found yourself in this situation, encountering some of these pitfalls and mistakes, dealing with neck and back pain that keeps coming back, don't beat yourself, don't blame your doctor or other medical professionals who haven't been able to help, and don't despair. Real change is possible. You can be free of chronic neck and back pain. There's no quick fix. But you will see more lasting improvement if you start addressing the underlying causes.

It won't happen overnight, and you may have some setbacks and exacerbations along the way. However, they will begin to happen less frequently, the episodes will be less intense, the duration of the pain will be shorter, and you will bounce back with therapy faster. I've seen it work for patients of all ages and with many different ailments, and I've experienced relief from my chronic pain. Treat the cause, not the symptom, and you will find your way to a life with less pain and more freedom to do the things you love.

CHAPTER 3

My Personal Experience with Chronic Neck & Back Pain

"It's not what you look at that matters, it's what you see."

Henry David Thoreau

My Struggle with Neck & Back Pain

I remember the first time I felt real neck pain. It was September of 1999 when I was 26 years old. My Penn State buddies and I were headed to watch the Penn State vs. Miami football game in Miami. Once we made it to Florida, we all crammed into an old college friend's apartment in Jupiter, FL. The lucky ones slept on couches. I had to sleep on the floor. The single pillow didn't help much. I woke up in the morning with a kink in my neck.

It was completely locked up, stuck to one side, and I couldn't get it to a neutral position. Plus, it hurt! A sharp pain stabbed at me whenever I tried to straighten it. I had never experienced an episode like this, and I was desperate for some relief. My recent graduation from physical therapy school gave me some idea of what was going on, so I coached one of my friends to press on specific muscles and parts of my spine.

That plus some over-the-counter pain meds helped alleviate some of the pain and free it up enough to go to the game, though I may have gotten a few strange looks for the way I held my head at a funny angle the whole time.

Over the next 13 years, my neck problems spiraled down a worsening path. My pain and dysfunction fell into three categories. The first was recurrent, episodic exacerbations that mimicked that first episode. The second was a constant tightness in my neck and the feeling that I needed to stretch or crack it. The third was a temporary neurological tingling sensation down one or both arms.

The episodic flare-ups were the most painful and debilitating of the three. My favorite medical diagnosis for this condition is "Acute Wry Neck." It's an old term, but it describes the condition well. They would usually strike without warning or apparent cause. Sometimes it would happen after waking in the morning, sometimes when I moved my head to look behind me. But it always came with a sudden muscle spasm, severely limited mobility, constant ache, and sharp pain during movement. For the first few days, the pain would be almost unbearable, but it would gradually subside into a manageable pain and a stiff neck that could linger for weeks.

At first, these episodes would happen once every few years. When I hit my 30s, they began to happen every year. Soon, I was getting them 2-3 times per year. One time I had a new episode before fully recovering from the previous one. You can imagine what that did for my mood. These flare-ups affect your quality of life in more ways than just the pain and reduced mobility. I can attest to the negative psychological effects of recurrent episodes over time that seem to have no rhyme or reason.

Between these acute episodes, my neck always felt tight and stiff, especially between my neck and shoulders, between my shoulder blades, along the sides of my neck, at the base of my head, and even in the front of my neck. Trigger points in these muscles would cause a constant, deep ache that would transfer pain to other parts of my head and neck. I had plenty of tension-type headaches and even started to get migraine headaches around the age of 30.

The other consistent feeling was that my neck needed to be manipulated or cracked. I also noticed that I could not tolerate static positions for long. Prolonged sitting or standing were aggravating. These problems weren't necessarily that painful or debilitating, but they were constant annoyances that I had to learn to live with.

The third symptom I often had was a numbness or tingling sensation in my arms and hands. They would come and go, but at their worst, I would wake up in the middle of the night with one or both of my arms numb to the point that I couldn't move them. It would only take a few seconds to a minute to come back to life, but it was a scary feeling. The tingling would also happen, albeit less dramatically, if I tried to hold a poor posture for a prolonged period, like when sitting in a car on a long trip or going for a long walk. Sometimes, they would accompany the acute flare-ups as well.

Though it may sound weird that a neck problem could make your arms go numb, the cause is simple. The nerves in your arms pass through the shoulder and neck on their way to the spine. When your neck is out of position, imbalanced, or misaligned, this can cause the nerves passing through this junction to become irritated, sensitive, or pinched, sending pain or numbness down the arm to your hands.

My back issues were similar but not as significant as my neck symptoms. Episodic flare-ups would occur in my back, though not as frequently nor intensely, and they wouldn't last as long. My back would tighten up and ache after prolonged sitting, driving, and standing. Like the neck, I would feel the need to crack my back for relief. At its worst, the pain would radiate down my leg into my groin, buttock, and calf. This often happened when I spent a day (or several days) teaching a course or giving lectures.

You might hear these different symptom presentations (acute flare-ups, intolerance for static positions with feelings of achiness and stiffness, and transient neurological symptoms) and think they were three separate problems. On the surface, that's true, and they might all require different treatments to manage and relieve when they arise. But for all three, the underlying cause is the same—a lack of optimal spinal and postural stability.

My Pain & Trauma Timeline

I learned about health life timelines from Danielle Raggi, the founder of the Pancafit Raggi Method.[8] The Raggi Method is a global postural approach aimed at postural rebalancing. This approach considers the

---

[8] https://www.pancafit.it/scopri-raggi-method/

patient in their whole, observing any parameter, sign, dysfunction, or trauma. An in-depth history timeline considers everything that has influenced a person's life and posture.

Here's my timeline:

Birth ---Age 49

Age 7	Neck trauma during a flip onto a mattress from a dresser landed on my head with my neck bent forward.
Age 8	Laceration of the right foot from jumping over a barb-wire fence around a garden.
Age 14	Bilateral Osgood Schlatter's disease (a common cause of knee pain in growing adolescents) lasted a year.
Age 16	Car accident, whiplash side-to-side, head impacted the passenger-side window.
Age 24	Hyperextension injury of left knee playing soccer.
Age 25	Onset of the neck and low back pain around the time I started working.
Age 26	First episode of significant neck pain (acute wry neck).
Age 28	Bilateral plantar fasciitis took around a year to resolve.
Age 28	Onset of regular headaches.
Age 30	Onset of daily and severe weekly headaches (diagnosed as tension-type and migraine headaches).

Age 38	Worst episode of neck pain while on a family trip to the Chesapeake Bay in Maryland.
Age 38	Significant left ankle sprain.
Age 39	Right shoulder injury during snatch in CrossFit (suspected torn labrum).
Age 42	Tooth infection and painful root canal.
Age 42	Onset of left hip pain and significant loss of mobility, unknown cause, took a year to resolve.
Age 43	Car accident that resulted in mild whiplash.
Age 44	Concussion from hitting horizontal support beam of playground set while yard trimming.
Age 44	Foot laceration from splitting ax.
Age 44	Neck trauma at Rehoboth beach. A wave crashed down on me while boogie boarding with my two boys. Slammed my face into the bottom of the ocean floor. I fractured my nose in three places and hyperextended my neck, leading to the inability to raise my left arm due to transient nerve palsy. Left arm weakness took 6-9 months to resolve. The left thumb and 1st finger numbness are still there on some minor level.

My primary problems include neck pain, headaches, and back pain. Secondary problems have been bilateral foot pain, hip and knee pain, and bilateral shoulder pain. Before my consistent neck and back pain onset, I'd already had two traumas in my childhood that may have predisposed me to later issues. The first time I recall having consistent pain was when I started a job at an outpatient orthopedic clinic in my twenties. Then came the initial episode of acute neck pain. By my late twenties, I started to develop consistent headaches, and at 30, I began to have regular migraine headaches.

My neck and back problems were at their worst in the decade between ages 30-40. To understand why, I needed to investigate stressful times and significant life changes during that time. I got married in 2004 (age 30). I left my job to start a private practice in 2005 (age 31). My two boys were born in 2006 (age 32) and 2009 (age 35). I worked on my post-graduate Doctor of Physical Therapy degree between the ages of 28 to 32. I taught, wrote, and presented at conferences between 2002-2015. I decided to grow the business and expand into a larger space in 2012. My dad died of lung cancer in late 2012, and my business showed signs of financial strain and decline beginning in 2016. Though not direct trauma like a car accident, these stressful situations can build up over time. I believe they contributed to my underlying dysfunctions that affected my body's physical health.

Make Your Pain & Trauma Timeline

Try doing a similar timeline for yourself. Recall when your pain problems first occurred and any significant traumas, injuries, or surgeries you have had in the past, whether you believe they are related or not. Here is how to do it:

1. List the top 3-5 major pain problems you have had over the years (back pain, neck pain, headaches, etc.).

2. Draw a line on a sheet of paper (a landscape layout will give you more room on the page). You may have to join several pages together if you have a long history. Write birth on the left-hand starting point and your current age on the right-hand end.

3. For each pain problem, mark on the line the first time you recall having that pain. Note the age and the problem above the mark. Do this for your top 3-5 pain problems.

4. Make a list of any significant, memorable injuries, traumas, or surgeries you have had in your past. This would include substantial sports injuries, falls resulting in injuries (such as hitting your head or cutting your chin that required stitches), car accidents, surgeries, painful procedures, etc. You can even include significant emotional traumas. If you have difficulty recalling past trauma, scan your body for scars or ask your parents or family for their recollection.

5. Mark those past traumas on your timeline as well. Note the age and the trauma below the mark. Do this for all your past traumas.

Now that you have your timeline, take the time to reflect on and analyze your history. This process will give you a better understanding of your pain problems and provide insight into the past traumas and injuries that may have contributed to the onset of your pain. Keep this list and add to it over time. Most of our lives are filled with painful, traumatic events, so don't feel bad about your list's length or significance. Instead, use it to help yourself and your healthcare practitioners get to the root causes of your problem.

3 Lessons from My Epic Boogie Board Fail

In July 2018, while at Rehoboth Beach for a weekend getaway with my family, I suffered a terrible (not to mention embarrassing) accident. I was happily boogie boarding with my two boys and family friends when a wave decided to pile drive my face into the ocean floor. It all happened so fast. I was in the wrong place at the wrong time. When I was able to come up to the surface and stand on my feet, I could tell something wasn't right. My left arm was limp. It felt like a sledgehammer had smashed my face. Blood was streaming out of my nose and mouth. My neck felt like it had snapped. I didn't choose to fight the Atlantic Ocean, but I did—and I lost.

The lifeguards checked me out. A medic assessed the situation. Amazingly, I was able to walk away. My wife and I decided to go to the closest emergency room. Six hours later, a CT scan of my neck, face, and head showed a broken nose in 3 places and a pinched nerve in my neck that had caused the short-term arm paralysis and the numbness and tingling of my left thumb and index finger. That was good news. It could have been much worse. A broken neck, paralysis, skull fracture, brain hemorrhage, a concussion, and possibly facial surgery would have been a much worse outcome. Whether through luck or a guardian angel, I made it out with relatively minor damage. Here is what you can learn from my embarrassment.

Acceptance

Accidents and injuries happen to everyone. What matters most is how you respond to them. In the ER, my mind was racing with negative thoughts driven by fear. Why me? Why now? How long will it take for me to recover from this? I tried to recognize that this type of thinking was not healthy. I focused on my breathing and felt grateful for not being worse off, even before knowing the CT scan results. If you become injured in an accident or suffer an injury that will affect your life, try to focus on accepting what has happened, find gratitude, and start to think of your recovery. Difficult as it may sound, it will be an immense benefit as you navigate a potential life change.

Immediate Self-Care

Do what you can to help yourself in the first few days after an accident or injury. I was cautious because my neck and face were swollen and painful, and I compensated throughout the rest of my body. I found positions of relief, iced my face three times a day, focused on breathing and meditation, took the prescribed medications, minimized compensations through walking, and started taking Bromelain, a supplement that helps with healing and cell recovery. Two days later, I was no longer taking the short-term pain meds.

The ER doctors told me to expect swelling and bruising within the next few days, but I didn't have any significant swelling or bruising, to my surprise. My self-care steps may have made a difference. When you get injured, it's easy to resort to meds and fear movement, but try to start doing whatever you can to help yourself recover. If unsure what you should or can do, ask a medical professional you trust.

Adopt a Positive Mindset

In the nine months before the accident, I had been practicing yoga, exercising, eating right, meditating, getting more sleep, and managing my stress. I am convinced that the immediate self-care steps and the positive lifestyle changes I adopted allowed me to walk away from this accident relatively unharmed. I don't think I would have responded or recovered nearly as well in the past when I hadn't taken care of myself and was more stressed out. But I know that the compound effect of positive lifestyle changes makes you more resilient and allows for optimal healing. A positive mindset can be powerful. It will help you focus on recovery and become more emotionally and physically resilient. Use it when recovering from any surgery or rehabbing from an injury. It beats the alternative of feeling miserable, victimized, and fearful.

I did undergo physical therapy as well, along with several self-treatment strategies on my own. The numbness and tingling are almost entirely resolved. Will I ever dare to enter the ocean and go boogie boarding with my kids again? You bet! The same can be true of your current or future pain, injuries, or surgery, if you remember these three lessons—acceptance, self-care, and adopting a positive mindset. It will serve you well.

My Interventions & Treatments

Whenever I tell these stories to my clients, they usually realize a few faulty assumptions they had made about pain and trauma.

First, many assumed that pain was an age-related phenomenon. In their minds, I was too young to have any significant chronic pain issues. Sometimes, they would initially question my understanding of their pain, thinking I hadn't lived enough to experience it. Though it's true that the longer you live, the more likely you will have to deal with pain problems, that doesn't mean a younger person in their 20s or 30s can't have a significant pain problem and a history of trauma that led to it.

Second, most assumed that because I was a physical therapist, I would have already addressed all my problems with physical therapy. Not true. You've probably heard that doctors make the worst patients. The same is true for physical therapists. Healthcare professionals expend so much of their time and energy helping others that they often don't have the time or the energy to help themselves, though this isn't good for the doctors or patients they treat over the long run.

However, my physical therapy education and experience did give me an advantage in helping myself. So, I started helping myself. At first, I did a lot of self-treatment to address my pain without relying too much on medications and medical interventions. I knew that treatment of my trigger points would help relieve the deep muscular aches and pains I was experiencing, so I did this at night or on the weekends. I also tried to practice good posture and have optimal body mechanics during work. I searched for that perfect pillow to get good sleep and addressed my over-pronated flat feet. I used ice and heat packs and rubbed my muscles with cream when necessary. All this gave me a short-term relief from some of the neck and back pain, allowing me to work and live more comfortably. And none of them take a physical therapist to accomplish. That's what I did initially to help myself, and I continue to do so today if I need to. You can also benefit from learning how to self-treat the myofascial components of your pain.

The self-treatment wasn't a permanent solution, however. Despite my efforts, the pain began to recur more frequently, and the techniques weren't as effective over time. I sought out other therapies and treatments. I saw a massage therapist from time to time. I started seeing an acupuncturist. I scheduled appointments to get treated by another physical therapist I knew and trusted.

All of it helped in some way. Massage therapy would relax my muscles, allowing me to feel looser and freer mobility. The acupuncture helped with the pain and rebalanced my energy. The physical therapy, especially the manual therapy and dry needling, helped restore my mobility and function along with the pain relief. I even went to a chiropractor to adjust my spine when needed. For acute flare-ups when the pain was high, I would take over-the-counter pain medication for a short time to make myself more comfortable. Everything helped a little.

But everything was also short-lived. My pain went down, I would be more comfortable, and my mobility would return enough to work and live, but the problems never truly went away. The reasons were twofold. First, my therapies tended to be very reactive. I only sought help when I was hurting and physically limited to the point that it hindered my ability to function and live. Secondly, I didn't do the therapies regularly enough to affect the root causes that would lead to longer-lasting change. Instead, I would do a couple of sessions, feel better, and move on with my life.

You may be wondering whether I ever saw a doctor about it, whether I got an X-ray or an MRI, and whether I ever considered surgery as a long-term solution. The answer is yes, yes, and no way!

I occasionally saw a primary care doctor when I had an acute episode that was so painful, constant, and uncomfortable that I needed a stronger anti-inflammatory medication. However, I can only remember one occasion when this was the case. I also got X-rays and an MRI of my spine twice, once after my worst neck episode and once after my trauma at the beach. The first round was more out of curiosity and to get a baseline of the structural changes in my spine. It showed exactly what I expected, some early disc degeneration, a narrowing of space where the nerves come out of the neck, and some bone spurs. This is entirely normal for most people my age. About three years later, after my beach accident, the second MRI showed worse findings of degeneration and dysfunction of my neck. I expected that, too, although it wasn't reassuring.

But those visits and scans weren't what helped me get to the root of my neck and back problems. They only confirmed what I already knew. And the answer wasn't surgery. Years before my boogie boarding accident, I had come to a more profound understanding of the real problem: my lack of spinal stability. Fixing that is what changed my life for the better. That didn't mean I was utterly problem-free (or immune to sudden beach injuries), but from that point on, the back and neck pain, which had been getting worse and worse, started to become less frequent and less intense, and I was more resilient to whatever pains and injuries did come my way.

Finding the Root Cause of My Chronic Neck & Back Problems

2013 was the year I finally decided to make the big changes I knew I needed. By that Spring, I felt my life had begun to spiral out of control. My business had expanded into a new space the previous March, so I was busy and stressed trying to grow my physical therapy practice. I was teaching more physical therapy courses than ever while also presenting at weekend conferences on dry needling and myofascial pain. My dad had been diagnosed with stage 4 lung cancer in the Fall, and he passed not long after, in December of 2012. My neck and back pain was worse than ever, and nagging injuries had forced me to give up CrossFit, my only form of exercise at the time, which I realized was doing more harm than good. I was overworked, stressed, and suddenly without many of the sources of support and escape that I relied on. I knew it was unhealthy, and I knew it needed to change.

I started practicing CrossFit in 2008. It fit the bill at the time. I needed to address the rising cholesterol numbers, poor energy levels, and weight gain that had resulted from working too hard for too long while neglecting my health. CrossFit allowed me a path to make that change.

I got in shape, became part of a community, and fell in love with Olympic-style lifting.

As a physical therapist, I knew it wasn't suitable for everyone, and I took care to focus on form and lifting within my capacity, at least during that first year. As time went on, however, I started going more often, maybe trying to do a little too much, and I got injured more often. Most of the injuries were minor until I suffered one shoulder injury at age 39 that was serious. It hurt like crazy, limited my ability to continue the workouts, and didn't get better for nearly a year and a half. But it turned out to be a good thing. My struggle to recover from that injury finally pushed me to understand the root cause of my issues and what it would take to fix them in the long term.

By the summer of 2013, after a ton of soul-searching, I was ready for a change. I wanted to exercise regularly again but didn't want to return to CrossFit. That turned out to be a crucial decision because, despite the turmoil I had been going through the past year, working out with a personal trainer introduced me to a positive influence that changed my life forever. The trainer's name was Pasquale Silvestre, but everyone called him Lino.

Lino is one of those larger-than-life personalities who positively affects everyone around him. We first met when I treated his shoulder at my physical therapy clinic. I loved our sessions. We talked all about human performance, health, and wellness. His knowledge and understanding of the human body were extraordinary. As an amateur bodybuilder, he had experience in human movement, functional training, and optimal performance.

As I was thinking about getting back to regular exercise and strength training, I knew I had to get stronger from the inside out. I had found that the traditional physical therapy approach to stability and strength training was not addressing my deeper spine stability issues. After talking with Lino, I knew I'd found the answer.

I reached out to Lino and asked to train with him. We spoke at length about my history of problems and my fitness goals. He agreed, but he wanted to do a few sessions of working on my posture and breathing before we started any training. I trusted him, so we got to work.

Those first several sessions were eye-opening. He worked on my diaphragm and my postural imbalances first. The first session on the Pancafit bench (a tool used in performing the Raggi Method) was incredible. I will never forget that session. It was a Friday morning, just before I left to teach a 3-day dry needling course in Virginia. I finished that session breathing easier, standing taller, and feeling more balanced and organized structurally. Even better, that feeling lasted through the three days of teaching. After a long day of teaching, I didn't get the typical nagging aches and pains in my neck and back. I was shocked in a good way. As a physical therapist, this approach was foreign to me. I'd never heard or seen anything like it in the US.

After several sessions working with Lino on the global postural approach, we started strength training at my office gym after work. First, it was twice a week and then went down to once a week. But these weren't your typical personal training sessions; I didn't lift any weights or do push-ups, squats, or lunges. Instead, he worked on my deep spinal and functional stability using the Dynamic Neuromuscular Stabilization (DNS) method from the Prague Rehabilitation School.

After a month, my aching neck, back, and shoulders, which had bothered me for a year and a half, finally started to feel better. I didn't need any dry needling, spinal manipulation, or other therapeutic interventions. I was floored. I knew we were on to something special.

Over the course of the following year, we slowly progressed my body awareness, movement coordination, functional stability, and functional strength. I spent most of the time on the floor, mimicking infant developmental positions, which are the hallmark of the DNS-type exercises.

It was a fantastic year of discovery and growth. It changed my physical health and functional ability forever. That spurred me to learn more about postural imbalances, fascia, and DNS. I sought out these courses, and I was hooked. As a result, I have been able to help many people who were struggling with similar problems. But the best thing I gained from that year was Lino's friendship. I'm forever grateful that he entered my life when he did.

My Introduction to a Global Postural Approach & Dynamic Neuromuscular Stabilization

The hour I spent on the Pancafit bench while Lino guided me to breathe, push, pull, and realign my body was my introduction to Posturology, a discipline that deals with the scientific and clinical study of posture. As a physical therapist, I'd learned about posture analysis in school, but this was the first time I'd heard about the Global Postural Approach.

My previous understanding of posture and postural dysfunction was basic. I understood that there are certain types of postural dysfunction like scoliosis (curvature of the spine), excessive thoracic kyphosis (rounding of the mid-back), and excessive lumbar lordosis (arching of the lower back), and forward head posture, to name a few. These are commonly seen by physical therapists, chiropractors, and massage therapists, and most patients have no problem recognizing them.

The typical approach to correcting someone's posture involves stretching the tight muscles, strengthening the weak muscles, improving a person's postural awareness and ability to correct their posture, and increasing their postural endurance. An attempt at lengthening muscles that are prone to being tight (e.g., hip flexors, chest muscles, etc.) and strengthening muscles that are prone to be weak (e.g., glutes, muscles between your shoulder blades, deep neck muscles) would usually involve individualized exercises that targeted these specific muscles groups, such as a hip flexor stretch for a tight hip flexor or resisted rows to strengthen the muscles between the shoulder blades.

One of the first problems with this approach is that it's strictly based on biomechanical principles. It doesn't incorporate the influence of fascia, the webbing of tissue that connects our skin, muscles, organs, and bones. Muscles don't function in isolation from one another. They are interconnected, like the links of chainmail armor, tied together through fascial planes or slings that run throughout the body.

Another problem is that strengthening individual postural muscles in isolation isn't how we learned to produce spinal and postural stability, to begin with, during our first year of development. And it doesn't incorporate the nervous system through our neuromuscular control. Spinal and postural stability is a synergistic sequence of motor control events that starts with creating intra-abdominal pressure, which then creates spinal elongation and further creates stability in other parts of our functional stability system, which creates the postural stability basis for the movement of our limbs. Thus, if we want to develop proper spinal and postural stability, we need to retrain these synergistic movement patterns with the same natural method we used during the first year of life.

A strictly biomechanical approach is also not sufficiently individualistic. We all share some consistent muscle and postural imbalances, but our unique genetics and trauma history create variations in our compensations that must be considered.

The biggest problem is that it isn't long-lasting. People will often come back to the clinic with the same problems despite having felt better at first. Consistent stretching and strengthening exercises will sometimes be enough to keep neck and back symptoms at bay. Still, most of us are not consistently doing the exercises once the pain has subsided and the initial urgency is gone. Plus, the exercises are often not the right type to improve their overall spinal and postural stability, which would provide permanent relief.

It is essential to free up the myofascial (soft tissue) restrictions and improve your joint mobility. It will relieve pain, free up your mobility, and improve your posture. Failure to recognize this critical component is why treatments such as spinal manipulation, manual therapy, massage therapy, and dry needling are effective for a time but don't maintain their effects for long.

Dynamic Neuromuscular Stabilization (DNS) is the glue that makes those treatments stick around for the long term. It is the best system available to address the underlying lack of deep spinal and postural stability. You must experience this stability for yourself to fully understand. You can feel the fundamental difference in your body and understand its vital importance to your optimal physical function.

The Global Postural Approach and DNS have become a mainstay in my practice. I still help my clients with manual therapy, joint mobilization, soft tissue manipulation, spinal manipulation, and dry needling, of course, but now that is just the beginning. Those techniques can relieve temporary pain and discomfort, but once I start addressing their postural dysfunction, teaching them about their breathing, and improving their awareness of their deep spinal stability, the real work and real change begins, just as it did in my own life.

CHAPTER 4

What Causes Spinal Instability

"There's so much gray to every story - nothing is so black and white."

Lisa Ling

Spine Anatomy & Biomechanics

To understand why people develop spinal stability problems, we first must have some basic understanding of the anatomy and biomechanics of the spine.

The spine is a set of bones, discs, joints, ligaments, muscles, fascia, and nerves. The bones that make up the spinal column are the occiput (head), vertebral body, sacrum, and coccyx. The vertebral bodies make up the bony, central part of the spine. There are seven of them in the neck (cervical spine C1-7), twelve of them in the mid-back (thoracic spine T1-12), and five of them in the lower back (lumbar spine L1-5). That connects to the sacrum; five vertebral bodies fused into one bone. The tailbone (coccyx) is at the tip of the sacrum. A rib cage of twelve ribs attaches to the vertebral bodies. Ten are attached to the front at the sternum, while the last two are floating.

Spinal discs are cartilage pads between each vertebral body from C2 down to the sacrum. A disc comprises two parts, the inner layer (nucleus pulposus) and the outer layer (annular fibers). The function of the disc is to add shock absorption.

The spinal joints are the junctions that connect the spine together, with one between each pair of vertebrae, between each disc and vertebrae, and connecting the vertebrae to the ribs, the ribs to the sternum, and the sacrum to the pelvis (sacroiliac joint). There are three types of joints in the vertebral bodies: the facet joints, the uncovertebral joints, and the costovertebral joints. Facet joints connect on both sides of each spinal level, providing the general mobility of the spine to bend forward and backward, lean sideways, and rotate. Uncovertebral joints provide lateral, side-to-side motion of the vertebrae. Costovertebral joints allow mobility of the ribs on the spine.

The sacroiliac joint allows mobility between the spine and the pelvis, providing a way to transfer forces between the lower body and the spine. The upper cervical spine is made up of the relation of the head (occiput), the Atlas (C1), and the Axis (C2). These joint articulations are unique in their shape and allow for the movement of the head on the upper neck. Fifty percent of our neck rotation happens between C1 and C2, so keeping this spinal segment mobile is vital.

Joints do not magically stay connected to each other on their own. They are held in place by cartilage and ligaments. This gives the joint complex some passive stability.

Nor can joints move on their own. They move when other forces pull on them, which is the job of the muscle and fascial system. Muscles attach to the joints through tendons, which allow for two main functions: stability and mobility.

Some muscles are designed to give stability to a joint. For example, the deepest muscles along the spine are called the multifidi. These muscles are layered, each covering three vertebral bodies, woven together to help stabilize each spinal segment.

Other muscles are designed to provide mobility. When these muscles contract, they produce forces that generate the larger movements of our trunk and extremities. For instance, the rectus abdominis (the front layer of our abdominals) allows us to flex our spine during a sit-up.

The multiple types of body structures (skin, muscles, tendons, ligaments, joints, bones) are interconnected by tissue called fascia, which is a type of webbing that can span large areas and is critical to creating form and structure within the body. Tight fascia can contribute to problems far from their origin. For instance, tight back fascia can influence how far you can raise your arms or contribute to plantar fasciitis (inflamed connective tissue in the sole near the heel).

None of this works without the nervous system. The nervous system sends and receives messages from the skin, muscle, and joint receptors to inform us where the joints are in space and enable control over postural stability and movement. In this context, motor control and coordination are primarily nervous system functions.

Structure vs. Function (Chicken or Egg)

Now that you have some basic understanding of anatomy, it is crucial to understand the difference between structural and functional approaches to muscle imbalances. Dr. Valdimir Janda (1923-2002), a Czech neurologist and physiotherapist, was at the leading edge of the science and clinical understanding of muscle imbalances. He observed two schools of thought in musculoskeletal medicine—structural and functional.

The structural approach is focused on the tissue structure as a source of musculoskeletal pathology. It is primarily rooted in understanding anatomy and biomechanics and relies on imaging (X-ray, MRI, etc.) to diagnose problems. Treatment is focused on immobilization, injections, surgery, and rehabilitation. Most orthopedic doctors take this structural approach.

The functional approach is focused on the altered function of the structural and physiological system as the source of musculoskeletal pathology. It is rooted in adequately understanding the muscles and their coordination related to other structures (bones, joints, etc.). In a functional examination, a clinician must visualize and understand the complex relationship of structures and design that are at play in the postural and movement system. The treatment is focused on addressing the pathology's root cause rather than solely on the pathology itself. Physical therapists are more likely to take this functional approach.

Looking at these differences between structure and function at the time was a massive paradigm shift in musculoskeletal medicine, and the medical profession is still working through it. These differences in perspectives are part of why patients often hear mixed messages from their doctors and physical therapists about their musculoskeletal problems.

For example, a patient with a disc herniation that irritates a nerve might hear from the orthopedic physician that their disc herniation, which is clearly visible on an MRI, is causing compression on the nerve and most likely leading to their pain. The orthopedist may tell the patient to try a conservative approach of rest, mediations, and physical therapy. They may recommend an injection around the spinal nerve if that doesn't work. If that doesn't work, then surgery is the only option.

But then that patient shows up at the physical therapist's office. The patient might hear that their problem is due to several body impairments and dysfunctions (e.g., poor posture, muscle imbalances, weak core, stiff hips, poor movement coordination, etc.) that have led to overloading of the spine, which ultimately led to the disc herniation. The imbalance between the load on them and their capacity led to sensitivity around the nerve. The physical therapist may say that the treatment will focus on several things to relieve pain and restore mobility initially but then will shift to addressing the root causes that led to the problem in the first place.

The orthopedist and the physical therapists have two fundamentally distinct understandings of the problem and how to solve it—no wonder the patient is confused.

So, which is correct? That's like asking which came first, the chicken or the egg. Does our structure determine our function, or does our function determine our structure? The answer is both.

Since everyone has a particular genetically determined anatomical structure, that structure will invariably create a specific pattern of functional postures and movements over time. The specific biomechanical forces that enable function also determine how those functions must be carried out in each individual. Also, pain-causing structural issues (such as an acute disc herniation irritating a spinal nerve) will cause someone to alter how they function to minimize the pain. If this continues for a long time, it will undoubtedly create new habits and modes of function.

On the other hand, your function will also influence your structure over time. The quality of an infant's development can majorly impact the rest of their life. So can the nature of everyday experience at school, work, or home, in sports or exercise or lack thereof, while eating or sleeping or lounging. Even the influence of minor aches and pains can alter the posture and movement of the body on a subconscious level. All these small and large functional influences will affect our structural makeup over time, inevitably putting stress and strain on certain parts of the body, which may lead to acute states of inflammation, spasm, and pain.

Ultimately, our function is a more significant determinant of future problems than our structure. The reason is simple. We can control and influence our function, which will positively or negatively affect our structure. It is not your natural body that is the cause of pain. Instead, living in an unhealthy, imbalanced environment induces your body to create pain to make you aware of the problem. This is a powerful tool. You can use it to understand and transform your body and life—functionally and structurally.

Genetic Predisposition

Genetic predisposition can strongly influence our spinal stability. There's no getting around it. Many of us can see it in our own lives. I often hear comments from my clients saying, "I inherited my dad's bad back" or "I have the same hunched upper back and neck problems that my mom suffered for years." There is no doubt that genetics influence spinal form and structure, whether it's a predisposition towards scoliosis or systemic joint hypermobility. Both can directly affect the spinal system and stability over time.

Every person has a particular genetic predisposition. Some are predisposed to being tall and lean, short and stocky, too stiff, overly flexible, etc. For physical therapists, observing these body type characteristics gives an impression of a person's capability to cope with physical stress.

The categorization of the somatic-type characterization was first described by German psychiatrist Ernst Kretschmer. In his book, Physique and Character, published in 1921, he attempted to show the relationship between body types, personality, and risk of mental disorders. He classified three constitutional body types: the tall, thin "asthenic type," the more muscular "athletic type," and the round "pyknic type."[9]

Dr. William Sheldon, an American doctor, psychologist, and follower of Kretschmer, researched the differences between these body types. He coined the term somatotypes and changed the names of the classifications to endomorph (round and soft), mesomorph (square and muscular), and ectomorph (thin and fine-boned). Sheldon stated that each person has a part of each body type, and that the individual should not be classified as one distinct body type. Instead, we all have aspects of each body type but varying degrees to one another.

He used a classification system between one and seven. A one meant the body type was hardly present, while a seven meant it was maximally present. For example, someone with an Endomorph of 2, Mesomorph of 1, and an Ectomorph of 7 would be described as a marked Ectomorph body type with a minor Endomorph component. The problem with this system is that it is purely based on visual observation and is subjective. However, methods have attempted to objectify the classification with body weights and other measures (skinfold tests, girth measurements, weight, height, etc.).

This body type classification initially looked at a person's psychological characteristics as it relates to their body type. Still, we can use the physical and functional characteristics to examine how they may relate to spinal mobility and stability. For instance, endomorphs tend to have a high level of joint mobility. In contrast, a

---

[9] KRETSCHMER, E. (1925). PHYSIQUE AND CHARACTER. HARCOURT, BRACE.

mesomorph has a low level of joint mobility, and an ectomorph has a moderate level of joint mobility. When it comes to endurance, endomorphs tend to have low endurance and stamina compared to ectomorphs, who have a high level of endurance and stamina. As far as strength is concerned, mesomorphs have a higher muscle strength capacity. Specific pathologies may also be more likely to occur in one body type over another.

In my clinical practice, knowing someone's body type and genetic predisposition helps me better understand the person's capacity. For instance, it gives me an idea of how to determine the dose of my interventions and advise my patients about their sports and life activities. I have seen many cases where a patient's body type was not suited for the activities they were participating in.

An extreme example is a 15-year-old girl who is systemically hypermobile and participating as the overhead head throw-in specialist on her travel soccer team. She came to me with significant shoulder pain and subluxation after playing in three games on a Saturday. The irony is that her joint mobility probably allows her to throw the ball a great distance. Yet, her lack of muscular stability around her shoulder is why her shoulder became overloaded. She had problems because the load exceeded her capacity. This is why many people will sometimes experience aches and pains even when they are not necessarily injured.

Knowing your body type allows you to understand why certain activities, exercises, or sports may or may not be a good choice for you.

Our Development in the First Year of Life

It is common to recognize that significant Neurodevelopmental Disorders can affect a child's function physically, mentally, and emotionally. The role of physical development in more subtle and less significant neurodevelopmental and coordination disorders, such as Developmental Coordination Disorder, is less commonly understood and appreciated. What is also less understood is the possible contribution of these developmental deficiencies and delays to future neuromusculoskeletal dysfunction later in life.

Neurodevelopmental disorders are physical, mental, and emotional disabilities primarily associated with the functioning of the brain and the neurological system. Examples of neurodevelopmental disorders in children include cerebral palsy, autism, attention deficit hyperactivity disorders (ADHD), intellectual disabilities (mental retardation), learning disabilities, and disabilities associated with vision and hearing impairments. Children with these conditions can experience various difficulties that involve learning, speech, language, behavior, memory, and motor skills.[10]

Developmental Coordination Disorder (DCD) are disorders that can interfere with motor skills and coordination. DCD occurs with a delay in developing motor skills or coordination difficulties that interfere with a child's ability to perform everyday tasks. The diagnosis is made

---

[10] UNITED STATES ENVIRONMENTAL PROTECTION AGENCY. (2015). AMERICA'S CHILDREN AND THE ENVIRONMENT: NEURODEVELOPMENTAL DISORDERS- THIRD EDITION https://www.epa.gov/sites/default/files/2019-07/documents/ace3-neurodevelopmental-updates_0.pdF

when the physical movement impairments can't be linked to another known physical, neurological, or behavioral disorder. DCD can affect the physical activities of everyday life such as getting dressed, handwriting, tying shoes, playing outside, and school-related gym activities. It is believed to affect 5-6% of school-aged children and occurs more frequently in boys.[11]

Children with DCD can present with broad physical, emotional, and behavioral difficulties, or only specific difficulties in certain areas. Leaving the emotional and behavioral problems aside, these are the most common physical characteristics of children with DCD.

Physical Characteristics of Children with DCD[12]

1. The child may appear clumsy or awkward in their movements. They may bump into, spill, or knock things over.

2. The child may experience difficulty with gross motor skills (whole body), fine motor skills (using hands), or both.

3. The child may be delayed developing certain motor skills such as tricycle or bike riding, ball catching, handling a knife and fork, doing up buttons, and printing.

4. The child may show a discrepancy between their motor abilities and their abilities in other areas. For example,

---

[11] MISSIUNA, C. (2003). CHILDREN WITH DEVELOPMENTAL COORDINATION DISORDER: AT HOME AND IN THE CLASSROOM.
[12] MISSIUNA, C. (2003). CHILDREN WITH DEVELOPMENTAL COORDINATION DISORDER: AT HOME AND IN THE CLASSROOM.

intellectual and language skills may be quite strong while motor skills are delayed.

5. The child may have difficulty learning new motor skills. Once learned, certain motor skills may be performed quite well while others may continue to be performed poorly.

6. The child may have more difficulty with activities that require constant changes in their body position or adaptation to changes in the environment (e.g., baseball, tennis, or jumping rope).

7. The child may find activities that require the coordinated use of both sides of the body difficult (e.g., cutting with scissors, stride jumps, swinging a bat, or handling a hockey stick).

8. The child may exhibit poor balance and avoid activities requiring balance.

9. The child may have difficulty with printing or handwriting. This skill involves continually interpreting feedback about the movements of the hand while planning new movements and is a challenging task for most children with DCD.

You may find yourself, your children, or your grandchildren encompassing some or all these physical characteristics. Before there was a medical diagnosis for it, it was often described simply as being "clumsy," "accident-prone," or "unathletic."

If significant enough, these physical impairments will be recognized by doctors and health professionals specializing in child development.

But it's often the parent or caretaker who spends the most time with the child who will notice a problem and bring it to medical professionals' attention. If the child is lucky, intervention and therapy will begin early. However, in my experience, unless the limitations are significant, this intervention rarely happens in the United States. When it does, it is usually for a limited time.

According to Pavel Kolář, originator of the Dynamic Neuromuscular Stabilization (DNS) method, children with central coordination disturbances caused by nervous system dysfunction can exhibit an abnormal model of motor behavior and positional reactions. This can influence general movement, but it also often leads to faulty body posture later in life with all the subsequent consequences on muscle adaptations.[13]

The DNS-influenced doctors, therapists, and researchers at the Rehabilitation Prague School believe that early intervention is necessary, even in those children who do not present with severe central nervous dysfunction such as cerebral palsy. Their system screens and identifies these central coordination disturbances in newborns and infants very early (within days or weeks of birth). This allows them to commence interventions that ensure the infant can develop as optimally as possible during the first year of life.

The physical development in the first of life is profound. The maturation of the central nervous system allows the baby to sense its

---

[13] KOLÁŘ, P. (2013). NEUROMOTOR DEVELOPMENT AND ITS EXAMINATION. IN CLINICAL REHABILITATION (PP. 100–101). ESSAY, REHABILITATION PRAGUE SCHOOL.

surroundings and undergo the postural development necessary to perform purposeful movements. The baby learns to prop itself on its elbows and lift its head. They learn to lift their head, arms, and legs on their back and start to reach for things. They roll on their sides and eventually on their hands and knees. They learn to sit, crawl, and kneel while remaining curious and purposeful in their desire to move. The maturation process continues for all gross and fine motor skills through ages of 5 to 6.

The quest to optimize a child's development isn't just about maximizing a child's physical potential to move. It is also about the postural development that results from these movements and their influence on the structural development of the spine, trunk, hips, shoulders, etc. The function affects the structure.

Therefore, it is doubly important to optimize the early childhood movement. It is necessary to monitor a child's developmental milestones, but not simply whether they have achieved a particular capability in a given time frame. It is essential to pay attention to how they have met those milestones and facilitate optimal movement quality.

Most of all, we must be careful not to negatively influence a baby's development with our desires to have them sit, stand, or walk before they are ready to. Keeping a baby off their stomach because it makes them cry is not good for their development. Propping a baby in a chair that allows them to sit before they have figured out how to do it alone is not good for their development. Placing a baby in a stander too early, before they have earned the right to stand, is not good for their development.

It may be hard to imagine that the subtle influence of parents and caretakers could significantly impact a child's development enough to predispose them to poor posture, poor movement patterns, and potential musculoskeletal problems in the future, but it can.

Too often, a reactive view of these childhood physical development issues is taken instead of a proactive one. We don't recognize the deficits until a child is not walking at 18 months after the negative impact has already occurred. The deficiencies in a child's development need to be recognized long before that point. We should learn from other countries, like the Czech Republic, to better understand and positively influence our children's development. We should give our kids the best opportunity to express themselves physically and minimize their predisposition for physical problems. The quality of how we develop and learn to move in the first year of life matters to our physical health.

Life Experiences

How we live our lives is another critical factor in developing muscle and postural imbalances that affect our physical capacity over time. The habitual postures and movement patterns we put ourselves through will affect the structure and function of our bodies. Like most anything else in nature, our bodies constantly change and adapt. We must recognize that physical habits, work activities, and our participation in exercise and sports is part of that equation.

Over many years, sports participation will influence our spine and postural instabilities. Gymnastics is a beautiful sport, but it does take a toll on developing young boys and girls. The repeated back bending and rotation involved in the sport can lead to spinal conditions like spondylolysis and spondylolisthesis.

Spondylolysis is a spinal condition when a crack forms in the bony ring on the back of the spinal column. This bone can fracture due to excessive or repeated strain, mainly due to backward bending and rotation movements. This condition is more prevalent in the young athletic cohort than in the general population.

Spondylolisthesis is a spinal condition where one of the spinal vertebrae slips forward over the one below it. This can be congenital or acquired and typically happens due to spondylolysis. The instability of one vertebra slipping forward over another can irritate the nearby tissues and nerves, causing pain and functional limitations. These conditions are more common in gymnastics, football, tennis, and martial arts. Children and adolescents are more susceptible because their spines are still developing, and the excessive and repeated strain can overload their spinal structures, causing weakness and spinal instabilities.

Work activities can overload the spine, leading to postural imbalances and spinal instabilities. Sitting at a desk for 6-8 hours per day will affect your posture, resulting in the hypermobility of certain aspects of your spine. Prolonged sitting is a major factor contributing to classic postural muscle imbalances that affect the upper and lower body.

That's why it is critical to have an excellent ergonomic setup and take breaks to minimize the ill effects of prolonged sitting and desk work.

Other work activities can affect the spine as well. Working on your feet all day or in a job that requires constant bending, stooping, or lifting puts a strong physical load on your body. If you don't have the physical capacity to handle the stress of a job, it will take a toll on your body. Over an entire career, it can lead to imbalances and loss of spinal mobility in some areas combined with hypomobilities and instabilities of other spine regions.

Daily habits have a significant influence too. Think about all the activities you do throughout the day. How do you physically eat, do the dishes, clean the house, do yard work, sit to watch TV, read, sleep, etc.? Do you walk around the house barefoot? Do you sit cross-legged at your desk? Do you sleep on your stomach?

These small physical preferences and behaviors affect our bodies over time. Just the fact of whether you are right-handed or left-handed makes a difference. Our side preference and dominance contribute to asymmetries and imbalances in our bodies. And don't forget about the influence of our psychological and mental states. Years of emotional trauma, anxiety, or depression affect our physical behavior. Someone who is scared, anxious, angry, or depressed looks and acts differently than someone who is not. If these states are consistent over time, they will become a part of our physical makeup.

Muscular and postural imbalances acquired from years of physical, emotional, and environmental factors will affect the load, stress, and tension on certain parts of our bodies and spines, predisposing us to future breakdown and injury. The blessing and the curse are that it happens slowly over time. No one habit or incident is debilitating on its own, but that also makes the problem hard to detect until it has become a serious issue. That's why it is important to recognize and address the effects of our everyday life experiences before it is too late.

Compensations Due to Pain, Injury, and Trauma

Injuries and trauma can have a devastating impact on our lives, and the effects stick with us long after the momentary pain has subsided, increasing the propensity for future neuromusculoskeletal problems. This is true for significant physical macrotraumas and microtraumas, surgeries and procedures, and even emotional traumas.

Physical macrotraumas include car accidents, fractures, and severe joint injuries. Subtle microtraumas might be rotator cuff tears, patellar tendonitis, plantar fasciitis, and recurrent neck or back tweaks. Surgeries and procedures can include orthopedic surgeries such as spinal procedures and tendon or ligament repairs but can also include non-orthopedic procedures such as abdominal surgeries and significant dental work. Acute or prolonged emotional traumas are events such as a near-death experience or a history of emotional or physical abuse.

All these things cause pain. Pain is a normal neurological response to a perceived threat and serves the purpose of self-preservation and protection. But prolonged pain can cause problems regarding our physical behaviors and movement patterns in the form of compensations.

When we injure ourselves or undergo a surgical procedure, the nervous system produces pain to alert us to take it easy and allow ourselves to heal. That healing process typically takes around 21 days for minor injuries and up to 8 weeks for certain types of fractures. The pain can be significant in the first few days, causing us to be guarded and protected. As time goes on, the pain subsides but may not be entirely gone, so we still aren't fully functional. If you have ever had an ankle sprain, you are probably aware of this phase when the significant pain has subsided enough to walk, but you don't feel like you can run or jump. The body is still producing pain because your tissues aren't completely healed, and your nervous system is alerting you that care is still needed before full participation in physical activities. This is natural. However, the problem arises in two specific circumstances.

One is prolonged fear and guarding. Some fear and guarding are expected early on, but if that fear of pain and guarded movement is prolonged, it creates abnormal movement patterns that can overload other body parts. The second problem is that some people have a highly sensitized nervous system which still produces pain even after the tissues are fully healed. This continued pain causes fear and anxiety, leading to a cascade of hormonal and metabolic reactions in the body that further produces pain, eventually leading to guarding and abnormal movement patterns. Both examples lead to compensation. Compensations can be subtle, even subconscious, and can go on for weeks, months, or years.

Example 1: Low Back Pain After a Bunionectomy Surgery

A patient came into my clinic complaining of gradual onset of low back pain of unknown cause, starting several months ago and progressively worsening. There is no history of recent trauma, injuries, or acute episodes. It seemed like the back pain appeared out of the blue.

Nothing ever appears out of the blue. My investigation during the history probed for any recent changes in their life. A new exercise routine, a period of decreased or increased physical activity, recovery from another physical problem, etc. The patient explained that she underwent a bunionectomy procedure a year ago because her bunion pain was no longer tolerable. She also didn't like how her big toe looked so deformed.

I knew recovery from a post-bunionectomy procedure could be challenging, so I asked her about it. She admitted that it was rough. She was non-weight bearing for a while, then she was in a walking boot for six weeks, then limped for quite a bit afterward. Walking with a boot can cause a considerable leg-length discrepancy if the other leg is not equally elevated with a heel or shoe lift insert. The compensation of walking abnormally for 2-3 months, along with her previous history of low back issues and poor spinal stability, eventually overloaded her back. Similar problems can occur with a person with flat feet or a past ankle sprain that was not rehabbed.

Example 2: Neck Pain After a Car Accident

Another patient suffered a significant whiplash injury to her neck during a car accident 15 years prior when she was in her mid-twenties. No one told her to do anything about it, so she didn't seek any help with rehabilitation. Once the immediate pain was gone, everything seemed to be fine except for a few things. Her head felt heavy, she had an intolerance for prolonged sitting, and her neck often felt stiff and like it needed to be cracked. She didn't think much of it at the time, but it continued to worsen over the years.

The whiplash injury was an acute trauma to her spinal segments, which usually affects the discs and joints of the spine along with secondary muscle guarding and spasms. The pain may subside over time as the body heals, but the movement dysfunction and increased muscle tension remain, especially since she didn't have any therapeutic intervention. This compensation continued for years and subtly affected how she carried herself and moved, contributing to further muscle imbalances and dysfunctional movement patterns. This stressed and overloaded certain parts of her cervical spine, leading to spinal segmental hypermobility. Therefore, she had trouble tolerating prolonged positions and holding her head up.

Example 3: Low Back Pain After Abdominal Surgery

A patient described onset of low back pain several months ago that seemed to come out of nowhere. She couldn't remember any trauma or injury. However, she did have a long history of low back pain, at least since her early thirties, and she recalled not tolerating sports as a teenager because it would bother her back. Other healthcare professionals had told her she was hypermobile and needed to strengthen her core. Also, she had an abdominal hernia repair a year prior. Her hernia wasn't terribly painful, but she was recommended to have it surgically repaired. She'd also had a hysterectomy three years ago.

Observation showed two scars related to her previous surgeries, and a physical examination revealed that her scars were not mobile and the fascia and connective tissue around them were tight. Further investigation revealed that she had poor breathing patterns, poor core activation in various positions, and hyperactivity of her back muscles with the movement of her arms and legs.

Several things could be at play here. First, abdominal procedures will result in some pain after the surgery. That pain will make people guard against excessive belly movement; even breathing could cause some discomfort. This is like a severe stomachache, where you might bend forward to try to avoid some of the pain. This guarding can alter how you move and breathe even after the pain has subsided. Another problem is the lack of scar mobility. Painful, tight scars not addressed therapeutically can result in limited mobility and inhibit optimal muscle movement patterns.

These examples highlight how the body compensates due to pain from injury and trauma and how that compensation can lead to dysfunction years later. These are just three examples; you can imagine the complexity of what someone's history of physical trauma could look like and how that might manifest later in life. However, not everything results in future problems. That will depend on the individual's load and capacity to bear it.

What is essential to understand and take away from this is that our body, especially our nervous system, is fantastic at compensating and will find new ways to move to avoid pain, even at the expense of optimal movement. Recognize this influence in your own life. Knowing that a particular body part may not have fully healed or recovered after that injury or surgery and that it may have altered how you move is crucial and should be addressed if you wish to function at your best.

Poor Body Awareness

Poor body awareness is also a predictor of future musculoskeletal problems. I have patients who have excellent body awareness and others who do not. When I teach them proper postural alignment or a coordination exercise, some people can easily and quickly demonstrate what they have learned in the next session. Others have a more challenging time learning new skills regarding their body's position in space and how to control the quality and speed of their movements. It may be due to a genetic predisposition, or some learned behavior, but it's relevant either way.

Our body is constantly talking to us about our neuromusculoskeletal system. We have all kinds of sensors in our skin, joints, and muscles that give us information about pressure, temperature, tension, etc. If we are more in tune with this part of our nervous system, we can better adjust to our surroundings.

For instance, nociceptors are nerve sensors that give information about chemical, mechanical, and thermal noxious stimuli. If you've ever sat on the toilet for too long, you have experienced the nociceptive alarm related to mechanical stimuli. It is a pain message that builds over time due to prolonged pressure on an area, telling you to move or change position.

What happens when we don't have good body awareness? We are less likely to receive the warnings and messages the body sends us, so we are less likely to make the necessary change. This could be due to disease or distraction. Diabetes, for example, can cause peripheral neuropathy, which dampens the nerve sensors in their extremities, resulting in dire consequences. A cut on the foot that goes unnoticed due to the lack of feeling, if it isn't cleaned or bandaged, could get infected and cause much more serious problems.

Poor body awareness can also manifest in more subtle ways. A distracted person who sits at the computer, intensely focused on their work, may ignore the messages that their back or neck is uncomfortable from the prolonged sitting in a non-optimal posture. Instead of changing positions, taking breaks, or properly supporting their postural alignment, they ignore the discomfort until it reaches a point that it can no longer be ignored. This leads to overstrained muscles and overstretched ligaments that compress the spine.

Over time, it can cause trigger point pain from muscular overactivity, ligament laxity, arthritic joints, and overloaded spinal discs that become weak, leading to disc bulges and herniations. The result is chronic neck and back pain of seemingly unknown origin because there were no major events, but the person failed to listen to their body's warnings.

The good news is that just as poor body awareness can be detrimental to your health, improving your body awareness will do wonders for your health. We call it multisensory integration. There are many ways to improve your body awareness because it is a multisensory system, including the visual, auditory, tactile, vestibular, and proprioception systems. Some improvements may require therapeutic intervention, but there are also many ways to learn how to train these systems on your own. Some practices you can do at home include meditating, practicing yoga or Pilates, learning a new physical skill or sport, or receiving massages. Activities like these get you in touch with your body's limitations and capabilities.

CHAPTER 5

Posture & Postural Alignment

"Some individuals may perceive their losing fight with gravity as a sharp pain in their back, others as the unflattering contour of their body, others as constant fatigue, yet others as an unrelentingly threatening environment. Those over forty may call it old age. And yet all these signals may be pointing to a single problem so prominent in their own structure, as well as others, that it has been ignored: they are off-balance, they are at war with gravity."

– Ida Rolf

Our posture reflects our disposition, our attitude. It's part of the persona we present to the world. We portray a confident attitude when we sit up straight or stand tall instead of slouched and slumped. When we adopt these good upright postures, it becomes our reality. We feel stronger, brighter, and more confident.

Posture is essential to our overall health. It is also often a reflection of how we have lived, so we can learn much from understanding our posture.

Posture affects our physical health through the biomechanical, myofascial, and nervous systems. Abnormal postural forces can increase compression, stress, and strain on our spinal structures, leading to degenerative changes. And our postural alignment influences the diaphragm's position, the lungs' ability to expand, and what muscles are activated, all critical factors in our ability to breathe.

Posture can influence our ability to stabilize our core, affecting our postural and spinal stability. The poor postural alignment will render a person incapable of stabilizing themselves. In contrast, correct postural alignment almost magically improves our core stability without thinking about or training it.

The influence of postural alignments on our breathing and stability means it inherently affects how we move. The most efficient and powerful physical movements in sport often go together with an optimal postural alignment. This is true with any sport, from tennis to Olympic-style lifting, downhill skiing to martial arts.

Posture can also affect our overall energy levels and our ability to maintain endurance with certain activities. Try sitting slouched at your desk while working at a computer for an hour. Don't be surprised if you feel tired and your back or neck is aching.

How can you improve your posture to maximize your health? Unfortunately, it's not as simple as sitting up straight or pulling your shoulders back. Changing our posture for the better requires the following:

- Restoring optimal flexibility of the muscles and joints

- Restoring optimal breathing

- Restoring optimal postural and spinal stability

- Restoring optimal postural awareness

Many health and fitness professionals aim to improve posture, including physical therapists, chiropractors, personal trainers, Pilates and yoga instructors, massage therapists, and bodyworkers. There are even methods specifically geared to improving postural awareness, such as the Alexander Technique and Feldenkrais Method. But not everyone will help you address all of the required factors.

Physical therapy can help address the many variables contributing to postural dysfunction and deviations. Physical therapy evaluations incorporate a postural assessment to define the severity of the postural problem, identify contributing factors, and recognize the relationship between someone's posture and their pain and dysfunction. Treatment of postural dysfunctions may involve regaining the optimal length of shortened muscles, mobilizing stiff joints, strengthening and endurance training of postural muscles, correcting environmental or ergonomic factors, and educating about postural awareness.

Once the postural influences of flexibility, breathing, stability, and proprioception have been addressed, the physical capacity for an ideal postural alignment is possible. But finding that proper balance is one thing; keeping it there is another. Education and awareness are the keys to long-term postural changes.

Just as your body has adapted to poor posture over several years, it can adapt once again to a more natural, ideal, and optimal postural state if you provide it with the right conditions. Remember that postural optimization spans our entire life. It allows a baby to develop the ability to sit, stand, and walk in the first year of life. It helps an adolescent who is going through growth spurts and body changes. It assists a middle-aged person in fighting the ill effects of a sedentary lifestyle. It aids an older adult who is struggling to stand taller and walk further. Regardless of where you are in life, it is not too late to experience the positive outcomes of improving your posture.

Fixing your posture isn't about perfection. It's about awareness, understanding its influence on your body and physical health, improving upon it, and maintaining it. These lessons will last a lifetime.

Optimal Postural Alignment

The ideal postural alignment places minimal stress and strain on the body while being conducive to maximum efficiency. When assessing your posture, you must compare it to this optimal postural alignment.

An optimal postural alignment starts with a stable base of support. The bones of the lower body should be in an ideal alignment for weight-bearing, the pelvis in a neutral position with the lower rib cage parallel to the pelvis, the spine upright, and the head erect in a balanced place over the chest.

Look at the optimal postural alignment from a side and back view (Figures 1 and 2). When evaluating a standing or sitting posture, we use a plumb line as a frame of reference. The body is centered on a fixed point from which we can measure deviations. In this case, that setpoint is the ankle and foot, as it will be a more consistent place to measure from than the head.

Side View

In a side view, the fixed reference point is slightly in front of the bone on the outside of the ankle. Here is an optimal side view using the plumb line as a reference. From bottom to top, the vertical line should be:

1. Slightly in front of the outer ankle bone
2. Slightly in front of the mid-line through the knee
3. Approximately through the outer bone of the hip
4. Approximately halfway through the trunk
5. Through the shoulder joint
6. Through the spinal bones of the neck
7. Through the lobe of the ear

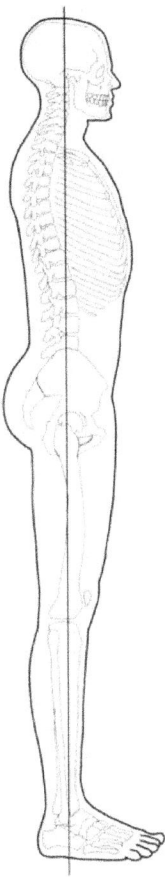

Figure 1: Optimal Posture (Side)

The ankle joints should be in a neutral position with the lower leg vertically straight and at a right angle to the foot. The knee joints should be neutral, not flexed or hyperextended. The hip joints should be neutral, not flexed or extended. The pelvis should be neutral, not overly tilted forward or backward. The lower spine should be slightly curved inward. The mid-spine should be slightly curved outward. The shoulder blade should be in good alignment and flat against the upper back. The neck should be slightly curved inward. The head should be in a neutral position, not too far forward or back, and not tilted forward or back.

Back & Front View

In a back and front view, the fixed reference point is halfway in between the heels. From bottom to top, the plumb line should be:

1. Halfway between the heels
2. Halfway between the lower legs and knees
3. Through the midline of the pelvis
4. Through the midline of the spine
5. Though the midline of the skull

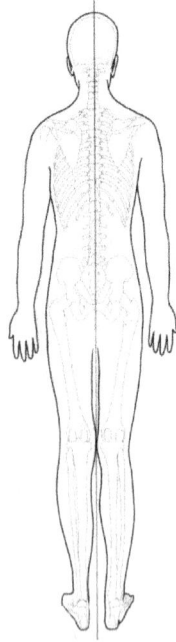

Figure 2: Optimal Posture (Back)

The feet should be parallel or slightly turned out, with the foot's arch in neutral, not overly pronated (flat feet), or supinated (high arch). The knees should be straight, neither bowed nor knock-kneed. The hip joints should be neutral, not overly aligned inward or outward. The pelvis should be level, not one side higher than the other. The spine should be straight, not curved one way or the other. The shoulder blades should be parallel to the spine and only a few inches apart. The shoulders should be level, without one higher or lower than the other. The neck should be straight, not bent to one side. The head should be straight, neither rotated nor tilted.

Clinicians who observe and assess posture will also look at the contours and shape of the soft tissues and muscles, not just the position or alignment of bones and joints. It's important to understand that no one has the ideal or optimal posture. You will find discrepancies and deviations from the standard. Our bodies constantly adapt and change by living life, and there will be inevitable postural deviations over time. However, it is beneficial to be aware of your postural deviations and how they correlate to your physical symptoms and how you feel. Keep in mind that these postural deviations can be improved upon over time.

Postural Faults

There are infinite ways for a posture to go awry, but there are a few more common variations. In assessing your posture, pay special attention to the pelvis's position and alignment, the position and alignment of the lower rib cage and chest, and the curves of the lower back, mid-back, neck, and head.

The pelvis position will simultaneously affect the lower back and the hips if the pelvis position is forward toward the toes or backward toward the heels. The tilt of the pelvis is also important. A pelvis tilted or rotated forward will cause more arching of the lower spine, while a pelvis tilted or rotated backward will cause more rounding of the lower spine.

The forces that act on the position and alignment of the pelvis are the hamstrings and hip flexors' flexibility (or lack thereof) and the relative stability and strength of the core, abdominal wall, and gluteus maximus.

The lower rib cage may be in a position that is elevated, which would lead to arching of the lower back and elevation of the chest and sternum, or it may be level or depressed. The chest may also be in a position that is more forward or backward relative to the pelvis, leading to a forward or backward-drawn chest.

The lower spine has a normal curve inward called lumbar lordosis, but an excessive curve (hyperlordosis) or a flattening curve (loss of lordosis) is possible. A normal outward curve in the mid-back is called thoracic kyphosis. The mid-back can also have an excessive curve (hyperkyphosis) or a flattening curve (loss of kyphosis or flat back). In the neck, there is a normal curve inward as with the lumbar spine, but an excessive inward curve is called cervical hyperlordosis, while the flattening of the curve is called loss of cervical lordosis.

The head may be positioned forward or backward in relation to the rest of the body, or it may be excessively rotated back or forward in relation to the neck.

Here are some common faulty postures:

Kyphosis-Lordosis Posture[14]

The hallmarks of this posture are the following:

- **Ankle Joints:** slightly plantar flexed
- **Knee Joints:** slightly hyperextended
- **Hip Joints:** flexed
- **Pelvis:** anteriorly tilted (rotated forward)
- **Ribs and Chest:** elevated lower ribs resulting in oblique diaphragm position and chest elevated
- **Lumbar Spine:** hyperextended (lordosis)
- **Thoracic Spine:** increased flexion (kyphosis)
- **Cervical Spine:** hyperextended
- **Head:** forward

---

[14] KENDALL, F. P., MCCREARY, E. K., & PROVANCE, P. G. (1993). POSTURE: ALIGNMENT AND MUSCLE BALANCE. IN MUSCLES TESTING AND FUNCTION: WITH POSTURE AND PAIN (4TH ED., PP. 69–90). WILLIAMS & WILKINS.

Notable imbalances:

- **Short and Strong:** neck extensors, hip flexors, and superficial low back muscles.

- **Elongated and Weak:** neck flexors, upper back extensors, abdominal obliques, and hamstrings.

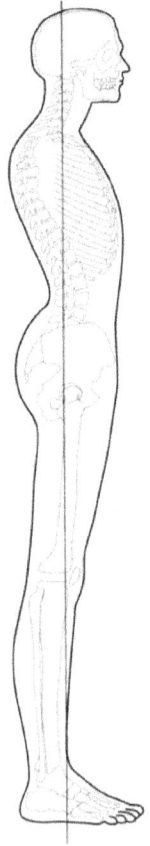

Figure 3: Kyphosis-Lordosis Posture

Sway-Back Posture[15]

The hallmarks of this posture are the following:

- **Ankle Joints:** neutral
- **Knee Joints:** hyperextended
- **Hip Joints:** hyperextended with the pelvis shifted forward
- **Pelvis:** posterior tiled (rotated backward)
- **Ribs and Chest:** elevated lower ribs resulting in oblique diaphragm position and chest elevated
- **Lumbar Spine:** flexion (flattening)
- **Thoracic Spine:** increased flexion (kyphosis) with upper trunk shifted backward
- **Cervical Spine:** slightly extended
- **Head:** forward

Notable imbalances:

- **Short and Strong:** hamstrings, strong but not short low back muscles.
- **Elongated and Weak:** hip flexors, upper back extensors, and neck flexors.

---

[15] KENDALL, F. P., MCCREARY, E. K., & PROVANCE, P. G. (1993). POSTURE: ALIGNMENT AND MUSCLE BALANCE. IN MUSCLES TESTING AND FUNCTION: WITH POSTURE AND PAIN (4TH ED., PP. 69–90). WILLIAMS & WILKINS.

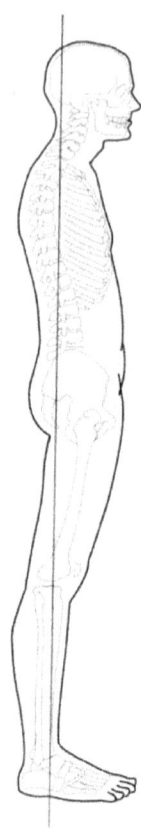

Figure 4: Sway-Back Posture

"Military-Type" Posture[16]

The hallmarks of this posture are the following:

- **Ankle Joints:** slightly plantar flexed

---

[16] KENDALL, F. P., MCCREARY, E. K., & PROVANCE, P. G. (1993). POSTURE: ALIGNMENT AND MUSCLE BALANCE. IN MUSCLES TESTING AND FUNCTION: WITH POSTURE AND PAIN (4TH ED., PP. 69–90). WILLIAMS & WILKINS.

- **Knee Joints:** slightly hyperextended
- **Hip Joints:** flexed
- **Pelvis:** anteriorly tilted (rotated forward)
- **Lumbar Spine:** hyperextended (lordosis)
- **Ribs and Chest:** elevated lower ribs resulting in oblique diaphragm position and chest neutral
- **Thoracic Spine:** normal curve and slightly shifted backward
- **Cervical Spine:** normal curve and slightly shifted forward
- **Head:** neutral position

Notable imbalances:

- **Short and Strong:** low back and hip flexors.
- **Elongated and Weak:** lower abdominals, hamstrings.

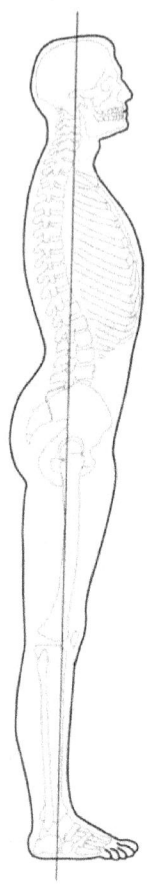

Figure 5: Military-Type Posture

Flat-Back Posture[17]

The hallmarks of this posture are the following:

- **Ankle Joints:** slightly plantar flexed

---

[17] KENDALL, F. P., MCCREARY, E. K., & PROVANCE, P. G. (1993). POSTURE: ALIGNMENT AND MUSCLE BALANCE. IN MUSCLES TESTING AND FUNCTION: WITH POSTURE AND PAIN (4TH ED., PP. 69–90). WILLIAMS & WILKINS.

- **Knee Joints:** extended
- **Hip Joints:** extended
- **Pelvis:** posterior tiled (rotated backward)
- **Ribs and Chest:** neutral
- **Lumbar Spine:** flexed (flat)
- **Thoracic Spine:** upper part flexed (rounded) and lower part straight
- **Cervical Spine:** slightly extended
- **Head:** forward

Notable imbalances:

- **Short and Strong:** hamstrings
- **Elongated and Weak:** hip flexors (iliopsoas)

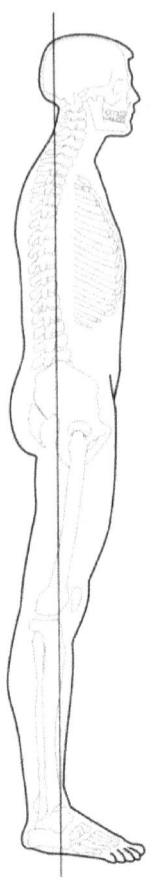

Figure 6: Flat-Back Posture

Posture Self-Assessment

You can quickly assess your posture by aligning your body against a fixed, straight surface. The best way to do this is to lie on your back on the ground or stand against a wall.

Posture Self-Assessment Lying Flat on Your Back

Lie flat on your back on a solid surface, legs together, arms by your side, and without any head support. Don't try to maintain any position; just let your body go and relax. Take note of the following:

1. What is the position of your head? Is it straight? Is it comfortable? Your posture may not be ideal if your head feels like it is extended backward or your neck feels compressed and uncomfortable.

2. What is the position of the back of your shoulders? Is there a space between the back of your shoulder and the surface? Your posture may not be ideal if your shoulders are not in contact with the surface.

3. What are the positions of your chest and rib cage? Do your rib cage and chest feel elevated toward the sky? If so, your posture may not be ideal.

4. What is the position of your lower back? Is it flat against the ground, or is it raised with space in-between? If there is space in-between, how much space? Is it uncomfortable or tight in this area? Your posture may not be ideal if your back feels arched, compressed, and uncomfortable.

5. What is the position of your knees? Are they straight? Are they contacting the surface? Your posture may not be ideal if your knee feels overly bent or hyperextended.

6. What are the positions of your legs and your feet? Are your feet splayed out with a separation between your legs? If there is, are you able to bring them together? How difficult is it to bring them together? Is it uncomfortable? Your posture may not be ideal if your feet and legs are far apart, and it feels difficult or uncomfortable to bring them together.

This same postural self-assessment can be done while standing up, using a flat wall as the reference.

Photographic Posture Self-Assessment

Taking pictures can help you get even more insight into your posture. Standing in your normal position, take photos of yourself from the front, back, and side. You can prop up your phone, use a tripod, or have someone else take the picture for you.

Be sure you aren't overly critical of yourself when looking at your pictures. Self-judgment is the worst kind of judgment. Very few people are pleased with what they see when I do this in my clinic. Most people have an idea of how their posture looks, but it's not uncommon for them to be surprised by what their posture looks like when they see the photos. Don't worry if it's not perfect. No one is. Instead, use this examination to learn more about and improve your physical self and posture. Here are some tips for taking your posture photos:

- Ideally, you should be dressed in your underwear, form-fitting athletic wear, or swimwear to see as much of your spine and body as possible.

- The area where you are taking your picture should be well lit.
- The background in your photos should be plain (a white wall is perfect).
- Be sure to stand with your feet together. The base of the big toes and the inside of the ankle bones should be touching.
- Pick a spot on the floor or the intersection of tiles to consistently stand in the same place.
- Photos should be full-body shots from head to toe.
- Stand in your habitual posture without trying to make any corrections.

What to look for in your photos?

The first thing to do is get an overall impression. How's your appearance? Better than you thought? Worse than you thought? What stands out the most? Where do you see tension?

If you printed out the photos, take the front and back views and draw a line through the following spots.

- Halfway between the heels
- Halfway between the knees
- Through the midline of the pelvis
- Through the midline of the spine
- Though the midline of the head

What differences do you see between the left side and the right side? Look at the size and symmetry of your legs, arms, and torso. Look at the alignment of your ankles, knees, arms, shoulders, and head. Compare your posture to the optimal back posture examples earlier in this chapter.

For the side view, draw a line through these points:

- Front of the outer ankle bone
- Slightly in front of the mid-line through the knee
- Approximately through the outer bone of the hip
- Approximately halfway through the trunk
- Through the shoulder joint
- Through the lobe of the ear

What differences do you see between the front and back of the body? Look at the alignment of your ankles, knees, shoulders, and head. Compare your posture to the optimal back posture examples earlier in this chapter. Do you align with any of the common faulty postures, Kyphosis-Lordosis, Sway-Back, Military-Type, or Flat-Back?

Keep these pictures as a baseline that you can compare to them at some point in the future. You can repeat them every six months to assess for any changes. An improvement or worsening of your posture is determined by the forces at play on your body over time. How you choose to live your life (exercising, minimizing sitting, adopting poor postures throughout the day, practicing yoga, etc.) will lead to either improvement or degradation. Outside environmental forces (recovering from a painful injury or accident, recovery from surgery, etc.) can also cause compensations that affect your posture.

Postural Correction

Now that you have a better view of your posture, you can start improving it. Correcting your posture is a dynamic process and a skill you must learn to ensure optimal spine health. For those with long-standing postural dysfunction, you will find correcting your posture difficult at first because your body is not used to maintaining a proper posture. The muscles and joints are probably not supple and mobile enough, and your nervous system is not attuned to the correct posture as the standard form of sensory input.

A stretching and spine mobility program will make this easier to attain, whether facilitated by a therapist or self-directed. By practicing the postural corrective procedures daily, your motor control and awareness will be improved steadily and dramatically. You can retrain your body and nervous system to get used to a better, more optimal posture.

Many people are looking for a quick fix. There are a lot of postural correction braces and devices on the market that promise to fix your posture. I have found that most of them don't work. They are too bulky and cumbersome to set up and maintain or don't induce the correct postural alignment. Many straps or braces make you feel that you are pulling your shoulder blades back, but as we have seen, that is not the correct postural fix.

Nothing compares in effectiveness to understanding and feeling the correct posture and how to maintain it for prolonged periods. It is difficult at first, but the awareness you gain in the process will help you make those changes throughout the day, day after day, week after week, month after month, and year after year.

Here are some simple ways to correct your sitting and standing posture.

Sitting Postural Adjustment Exercise

Step 1:

Start with your feet flat on the ground. If possible, adjust the height of your chair so that your hip is slightly higher than the level of your knees. Use a footrest if your legs are short and your feet are no longer touching the ground.

Step 2:

Now find pelvic neutral. Tilt your pelvis back to assume a slouched, rounded lower back posture. You should feel that the front of your body is coming together (ribs to pelvis) and a stretch in your lower back. Notice how this also affects your neck and shoulder position. Now tilt your pelvis all the way forward so that your lower back is arched and you feel a stretch in your abdomen (ribs and pelvis moving apart). Notice how this overcorrected position affects your lower back, neck, and shoulder. Now let go of that overcorrection until you feel comfortable. This is your neutral pelvis position. You should feel that you are sitting on your sit bones. You can place your hands under your butt and go through this same adjustment exercise to feel the movement of your ischial tuberosity (sit bones) and the stable pelvis position when you are stacked on top of them.

Step 3:

Ensure parallel position of your lower rib cage over your pelvis. Ideally, the lower rib cage and pelvis lines should be parallel. This ensures the optimal function of the diaphragm for its respiratory and stabilization functions. A quick or prolonged exhalation will ensure that you are in this lower expiratory position of your lower rib cage. Try blowing air out of your mouth through pursed lips quickly or slowly during a prolonged exhalation. Either way, you should feel a lowering of your lower rib cage. The result should feel like your trunk or core is integrated between your rib cage and pelvis. You should feel as though it is easier to breathe into your belly.

Step 4:

Correct your shoulder blade position. Put your shoulder blades in the optimal position by shrugging your shoulders upward towards your ear, rotating them back, and gently dropping them down. It should feel like your shoulder blades are back and down, sitting on your rib cage. Arms should be resting by your side.

Step 5:

Correct your head position. The last step is gently tucking in your chin slightly without changing the pelvis, rib cage, or shoulder position.

You should feel like you are elongating your head with the back of the head gliding upward and the chin gliding downward.

Step 6:

Learn to maintain these three natural curves in your back to distribute stress evenly on your spine while sitting for a prolonged period at your desk or computer, while driving, or while eating at a table. Use lumbar support to accomplish this. I recommend the Medic Air Pillow or the McKenzie Super Roll, depending on your body type and the shape and size of the chair. You can use a rolled-up towel, cushion, or piece of clothing as a substitute in a pinch.

Standing Postural Adjustment Exercise

Step 1:

Start with awareness around your feet. Place your feet shoulder-width apart. Distribute your weight evenly between your two feet. Think of stepping on two scales with both feet, so your weight distribution is the same on each leg.

Step 2:

Distribute the weight evenly through all four corners of each foot. Shift your weight forward towards your toes. Feel what muscles become more active in your body and how your body compensates. Now shift your weight back toward your heels. Feel how your body compensates here and what muscles are more active. Now find the neutral position of the feet so that it feels like you have evenly distributed weight in all four corners of your feet.

Step 3:

Knee alignment. Keep your knees straight or slightly bent, not hyperextended.

Step 4:

Find a neutral pelvic position as in the sitting exercise. You will find that your pelvic mobility (your ability to tilt your pelvis forward and backward) will be more limited. This is due to the length of your hip flexors and hamstrings, which are not in play while seated.

Step 5:

Align your rib cage over your pelvis (as described in the previous exercise).

Step 6:

Correct your shoulder blade position (as described above).

Step 7:

Correct your head position (as described above).

Step 8:

Keep your back straight while maintaining the natural curves of your spine. Find your steady lower belly breath in this corrected standing position.

Stacking the Blocks

Imagine stacking blocks on top of one another to build a tall tower. To erect a tall, stable tower, you would have to stack the blocks on top of one another as perfectly aligned as possible. Now imagine that your body is made up of the separate blocks of your feet, pelvis, chest, and head.

Sitting Correction by Stacking the Blocks

> If you sit with your feet flat on the ground or a footrest, find your neutral pelvic position as described above. Your pelvis is the bottom block, the foundation. Now stack your chest on top of your pelvis. Finally, stack your head on top of your chest. The result is an erect sitting posture. Ribs in a downward position parallel to your pelvis will ensure optimal diaphragmatic breathing and stabilization function. If you will be sitting for a long time, use lumbar support to help maintain the neutral pelvis position.

Standing Correction by Stacking the Blocks

> Start with your feet. Sway your body back-and-forth and side-to-side until you feel that the block made up of your feet is resting in its most stable, centered position. Now bring your attention to your pelvis and stack your pelvis on top of your feet. Now stack your chest on top of your pelvis. Finally, stack your head on top of your chest without changing the previous stacked blocks. The result is an erect standing posture. Carry this feeling with you throughout your day to improve your postural awareness.

Sitting or Standing Postural Correction using String Pull to the Sky

Another quick way to correct your posture is to imagine a line of string pulling you up from the crown of your head. Sit or stand and imagine a piece of string attached to the top of your head is pulling upward. Imagine elongating your spine in one fluid motion without hyperextending through your lower back, lifting your chest, or extending your neck. This is a quick correction you can even do while walking.

CHAPTER 6

Breathing

"The body is solid material wrapped around the breath."

Dr. Ida Rolf

"If breathing is not normalized, no other movement can be."

Dr. Karel Lewit

Importance of Optimal Breathing

What is the most significant change you can make to improve your overall health and physical well-being? Improve your breathing capacity and ability. Restoring and optimizing the respiratory function of the diaphragm (your breathing muscle) is the most impactful change a person can make to their physical health. It can also be valid for improving spiritual, mental, and emotional health since it relates to quieting the mind and finding stillness through meditation and other similar practices.

Why is optimal breathing so impactful? Quite simply, without breath, there is no life. Outside of that obvious fact, the quality of our breath is critical to the proper functioning of all our body's systems. Every system in our body relies on oxygen—the respiratory system, the cardiovascular system, immune system, digestive system, etc. Optimizing your breath can help with a wide array of physical functions, from more efficient digestion of food to improved immune response, from managing your blood pressure to increasing your cognitive abilities.

Some healthcare and wellness professionals blame poor breathing habits and their secondary consequences on many widespread ailments and diseases. Abnormal respiratory patterns are referred to as Breathing Pattern Disorders. Respiratory therapists, physical therapists, pulmonologists, yoga instructors, and many other healthcare professionals aim to restore optimal breathing patterns to facilitate health and wellness goals.

Hyperventilation is an example of an extreme breathing pattern disorder. You can think of ideal breathing on one end of the spectrum and hyperventilation on the other. Although hyperventilation is not usually a chronic or constant state for most who suffer from it, a milder version may be more common than you think.

Many of us take shallow breaths high in our chest that is too quick and inefficient—a milder version of hyperventilation. In essence, most of us are over-breathing much of the time. This type of shallow breathing pattern causes the carbon dioxide (CO_2) concentration levels to be too low, changing the pH of our blood to become too alkaline and causing respiratory alkalosis. This is called Hypocapnia. It has been hypothesized that hypocapnia is a significant contributing factor in many chronic diseases such as heart disease, high blood pressure, chronic pain, anxiety, lack of energy, poor posture, and low back and neck conditions.

One side-effect of hypocapnia is smooth muscle constriction, which causes blood vessel constriction and gut narrowing. Another is the loss of calcium in the urine, which causes muscles and nerves to function poorly. The physical effects include exhaustion, tingling, cramps, weakness, and irregular blood flow. The psychological effects are fatigue, sensitivity to light and sound, and dizziness.

The kicker is that these symptoms create fear and anxiety, causing the body to go into a sympathetic nervous system drive state (fight or flight response), which leads to even more upper body tension and poor breathing patterns. Dr. Lum (1975), a pulmonologist, describes this vicious cycle of poor breathing habits:[18]

> *It has always seemed to me that hyperventilation is essentially a bad habit, a habit of breathing in such a way that the day-to-day level of CO2 is relatively low. Given this basic bad habit, any physical or emotional disturbance may trigger off a chain reaction of increased ventilation, rapidly producing*

---

[18] CHAITOW, L., GILBERT, C., BRADLEY, D., & CHAITOW, L. (2014). WHAT ARE BREATHING PATTERN DISORDER? IN RECOGNIZING AND TREATING BREATHING DISORDERS: A MULTIDISCIPLINARY APPROACH (SECOND, P. 4), CHURCHILL LIVINGSTONE.

hypocapnia symptoms, alarm engineered by the symptoms, consequent sympathetic arousal resulting in increased ventilation and increased symptoms.

Breathing pattern disorders tend to be underrated and underdiagnosed and thus are not being adequately addressed for many people who suffer from their ill effects.

Although breathing pattern disorders can affect many physical systems like our cardiovascular system, metabolic systems, and psychological states like anxiety; much of this won't be discussed in this book. My primary focus in this chapter is to describe the impact of improving your breathing capacity and diaphragmatic function on your postural and spinal stability and how that can positively impact chronic neck and back pain. The beautiful thing is that improving your breathing capacity and diaphragmatic function will positively benefit many other aspects of your physical and psychological health and well-being in addition to your postural and spinal stability.

Anatomy and Function of Breathing

To better understand breathing and how to improve it for ourselves, we must appreciate its anatomy and function first. Breathing is the exchange of gasses housed in a skeletal system through muscles that contract and relax, controlled by the nervous system.

Skeletal System

Let's start with the skeletal system (the bones and joints) involved in breathing. Many bones and joints provide a stable, flexible structure that allows for considerable mobility and acts as a framework for the muscles involved with breathing.

The first thing to note is the thoracic cage, which consists of more than 80 joints. The back is made up of the twelve thoracic spinal vertebrae and the ribs that attach to each of them in the back. The vertebrae's connection to the ribs is called a costovertebral joint. There are twenty-four joint connections in total, twelve on each side.

The ribs wrap around the sides and attach to costal cartilage in the front, which connects to the sternum. This connection from front to back creates a costal arc at each level capable of mobility.

The ribs are bony structures but part of a flexible unit because of their attachments, making them elastic and deformable. That's a good thing. They can expand and return to their original shape, bending and twisting as needed.

The suppleness of the elastic cartilage adds to the mobility of the ribs at the point of attachment to the spine and the sternum. This mobility can diminish due to aging and decreased mid-back mobility, but it also can be improved through deliberate training. So, it's imperative to improve and maintain the mobility of the spinal column, particularly the thoracic spine, to optimize your breathing capacity, posture, and spinal stability.

Respiratory Organs

The lungs are the active organ of respiration. They are located in the upper half of the rib cage; the right lung is larger than the left. The primary function of the lungs is the gas exchange of oxygen and carbon dioxide in and out of our bloodstream. The lungs transfer oxygen from the air we breathe to our arterial bloodstream, sending it to the left side of the heart and out to the body. The venous bloodstream returns the blood from the body back through the right side of the heart to the lungs, where the carbon dioxide-rich blood is transformed into oxygen-rich blood. Each lung has tiny sacs containing pulmonary alveoli (approximately 300 million of them!), where oxygen and carbon dioxide exchange occurs.

Pleura membranes wrap around the inner and outer layers of the lungs. The outer layer of this pleura attaches to the ribs and diaphragm. The lungs adhere to the thorax, so the movement of the diaphragm and ribs affect the lungs and vice versa.

The air we breathe is transported through two channels: the inferior and superior airways. The superior airway passage lies above the thorax and is made up of the nose, the mouth, the pharynx, the larynx, and the trachea. This system is flexible, adapting to movements of the head and neck during breathing. Air can be inhaled through the nose or mouth. Air inhaled through the nose passes through three levels of the pharynx (nasopharynx at the top, oropharynx at mid-level, and laryngopharynx at the bottom). Air inhaled through the mouth only passes through the bottom two levels. The larynx is connected at the top to the pharynx and sits atop the trachea. The larynx is a sphincter that allows air to pass through and is also where we produce sound through our vocal cords. The last piece of the superior airway passage is the trachea, an accordion-like airway passage that extends from the larynx to the primary bronchi at the bottom.

The inferior airway passage comprises the bronchi (shaped like a pipe). The two primary bronchi run from the trachea to the lungs and diverge into secondary bronchi, which run to each lobe of the lungs. The bronchi then divide each lobe into bronchioles and then split further into smaller bronchioles until they branch into alveolar ducts. The entire structure looks like an inverted tree with many splintering branches.

Respiratory Muscles

Many different muscles can act on or influence our breathing. Some muscles assist with inspiration (breathing in) and others with expiration (breathing out). Some muscles help with both. Most of these muscles' influence on breathing is not their only primary function but a secondary one. The most influential muscle that acts on our breathing is the diaphragm.

Muscles of inspiration help increase the volume of the lungs by expanding the lungs through a pulling action at the base and outside surfaces of the lungs.

The diaphragm is one of our body's most unique and fascinating muscles. There is no other muscle quite like it. Its primary responsibility is for our regular, involuntary breathing. It acts like a pump or a piston for the lungs. It also has an essential secondary function in spinal and postural stability, which I will discuss further in the next chapter.

The diaphragm is a large, thin, fibrous muscle that connects the thorax and the abdomen. It is shaped like a large dome closely situated between the organs and flexible in form. The right side of the diaphragm is slightly higher than the left, possibly since the organs on the right-hand side of our abdomen take up more space.

The anatomy of the diaphragm is one of the reasons it is so fascinating. At the diaphragm's center is a fibrous part called the central tendon, where the muscle fibers of the diaphragm are attached in a circular fashion. The muscle fibers flare out and join the circumference of the rib cage, thus giving it a dome-like shape. From the central tendon, it attaches to the back part of the xiphoid process (bottom tip of the sternum), the inside part of the lower ribs, the rib cartilages (ribs 7-12), and the upper part of the lumbar spine (L1-3).

When the diaphragm contracts, it flattens downward toward the abdomen and pelvis, which indirectly lifts and pushes the ribs apart. It essentially acts as a piston between the thorax and abdomen. But unlike some of our muscles, it doesn't have much sensory innervation, so its contraction is challenging to perceive. That's one reason people have difficulty training it.

Another fascinating aspect of the diaphragm is that its motor innervation (nerve control) is from the phrenic nerve, which stems from C3-5. That means its neural input comes from the neck. It has three openings that allow certain structures to pass between the thorax and the abdomen. These openings are the esophageal opening for the esophagus and the vagus nerve (control of the digestive system), the aortic opening for the aorta (body's main artery that transports blood from the heart), and the thoracic duct (main vessel of the lymphatic system), and the caval opening for the inferior vena cava (large vein that transports blood to the heart). The muscle also closely connects to the lungs and the abdominal organs. Every time the diaphragm moves, it influences the lungs above and the abdominal organs below, affecting their shape and function.

Other muscles of inspiration include muscles that lift or open the rib cage from the outside, whereas the diaphragm does so from the inside. These muscles include the pectoralis (ribs-to-shoulder-girdle muscle), the serratus anterior (ribs-to-shoulder blade muscle), the serratus posterior superior (ribs-to-spine muscle), and the scalene and sternocleidomastoid (ribs-to-head/neck muscles). These muscles are called accessory breathing muscles and are primarily superficial. They mainly aid in lifting the rib cage for maximum expansion, which is not necessary for normal breathing at rest but may be helpful during physical activity and exertion or may be overactive in a compensatory fashion.

Muscles of expiration act to increase the expiratory reserve volume and the force and rate of exhalation. They assist in reducing the volume in the lungs by dropping the ribs, raising the base of the lungs, or both. Like the muscles of inspiration, these muscles have other functions outside of assisting with respiration since the first and primary expiration force is due to the elasticity of the lungs recoiling, which is responsible for much of our normal exhalation.

Muscles of expiration include the abdominal muscles (rectus abdominis, transverse abdominis, and internal/external obliques). The rectus abdominis lies superficially in the front (the six-pack muscle), attaching between the lower front rib cage and sternum to the pubic bone. The transverse abdominis is the deepest layer in the lower abdomen that attaches to the lumbar spine, pelvis, inguinal ligament, and thoracolumbar fascia (the connective tissue that connects to our back). The internal and external obliques are diagonally oriented abdominal muscles that attach between the lower rib cage to the pelvis and inguinal ligament. Other muscles that can be involved in expiration are the transversus thoracics (inside the rib cage), the quadratus lumborum (an important back muscle that attaches from the twelfth rib to the pelvis and spine), and the serratus posterior inferior (a muscle that runs between the lower thoracic and upper lumbar spine to the lower ribs).

The internal and external intercostals are the final set of muscles involved in respiration. These are the muscles that lie in between each rib. Their action depends on whether the ribs are fixed downward or upward. If the ribs are fixed upward, the intercostals will pull the ribs upward (inspiratory function). Conversely, the intercostals will pull the ribs downward (expiratory function) if the ribs are fixed downward. So, they can assist in both inspiration and expiration.

Neural Regulation of Breathing

The autonomic nervous system controls the neural regulation of our internal organs and is responsible for the unconscious maintenance of our internal body environment. In addition to breathing, it regulates our blood pressure, heart rate, body temperature, digestion, metabolism, and bowel and bladder functions.

The respiratory center lies in the most primitive part of our brain, the brainstem. It automatically adjusts ventilation to maintain arterial blood oxygen and carbon dioxide pressures at a constant level that sustains the proper internal environment necessary to support life. If there is a chemical imbalance of oxygen or carbon dioxide concentrations, the sensory aspects of the respiratory center will respond accordingly to regain this balance. Even though that breathing is mainly automatic, it can be influenced and overridden by conscious effort. This voluntary control can be beneficial, as when we use our breath to yell or sing. But it can also be unhelpful, as with the shallow breathing that accompanies chronic states of mental anxiety.

Optimal Breathing Pattern

Breathing Development

To understand an optimal breathing pattern, we must appreciate how our breathing functionality developed, starting at birth. At birth, the baby has an immature central nervous system, and therefore has undeveloped breathing, muscle, movement, and sphincter function. As the central nervous system develops, so does its breathing, posture, and movement ability. By 4-5 months, an infant can coordinate breathing with vocalization, and costal breathing is fully established by 6 months.

Postural Considerations

For optimal breathing to occur, the spine and rib cage must have a flexible, compliant, and functional structure. This includes both the skeletal and soft-tissue components. If there are postural restrictions, the rib cage will not respond appropriately to the muscular forces acting on them, inhibiting the rise and fall of the chest, altering the oxygen levels in the blood, and leading to compensations, which will eventually produce non-optimal breathing function. Therefore, attention to posture is essential to breathing well.

Postural faults can be a problem for optimal breathing because they affect the function of the diaphragm. Ideally, the alignment of the rib cage should be parallel to the alignment of the pelvis. This allows the diaphragm to lie in a horizontal plane so that it can contract downward toward the pelvis when it contracts. This diaphragm contraction is involved in a force couple with the pelvic floor, allowing the diaphragm to function as a piston and maximizing the rib cage's ability to move, which increases lung volume. This is the physical manifestation of the respiratory system's ideal biomechanical function. As you will see in the next chapter, it is also the basis of optimal spinal and postural stabilization.

What parameters make up an optimal breathing pattern?[19]

- Efficient movement of oxygen and carbon dioxide in and out of the lungs to meet the metabolic demands of the body
- The ability of the diaphragm to contract and descend into the abdominal area during inhalation, expanding the rib cage outward and upwards during involuntary, quiet breathing
- The ability of the diaphragm to return to its relaxed position during exhalation
- A respiratory rate of 10-14 breaths per minute
- A ratio of inspiration to the expiration of 1:1.5-2
- Efficient and least amount of mechanical effort of the respiratory muscles

How Does an Optimal Breathing Pattern Look?

Babies often give the best example of an optimal breath pattern. If you observe a baby in a relaxed posture on their back, you will see the following:

The first thing to move during inspiration is the belly. The stomach expands outward in all directions. At the end of inspiration, there is a slight expansion of the upper ribs and chest. This is due to the downward movement of the diaphragm towards the pelvis as it

---

[19] Chaitow, L., Gilbert, C., Bradley, D., & Chaitow, L. (2014). The Structure and Function of Breathing. In Recognizing and Treating Breathing Disorders: A Multidisciplinary Approach (Second, p. 4), Churchill Livingstone.

contracts on inhalation. The expansion of the rib cage results from the inflation of the lungs.

Next, the lower rib cage expands outward in all directions, and the upper rib cage expands upward toward the end of the inhalation phase. If you put your finger between their ribs, you would feel the spaces between them widen. The sternum moves along a forward and backward plane. The diaphragm is horizontally situated (in an upright posture) and parallel in relation to the pelvis. The excursion of the diaphragm is full and sufficient. Their breath is easy and accessible without much effort, and there is no visible contraction of any superficial muscles of the head and neck.

The optimal breath pattern at rest is called diaphragmatic breathing, also known as abdominal or stomach breathing. Here's how the diaphragm works during inhalation. The attachments of the diaphragm are relatively fixed around the circumference of the rib cage, while its attachment to its central tendon is mobile. As it contracts, the central tendon gets pulled toward the pelvis. This descent of the diaphragm influences the base of the lungs above, ultimately creating a negative pressure or vacuum, which makes up the inhalation phase. The diaphragm movement downward also affects the contents below the diaphragm, creating an inflation effect on the abdominal wall. Most observe this as the outward expansion of the abdomen, hence the notion of breathing through the stomach.

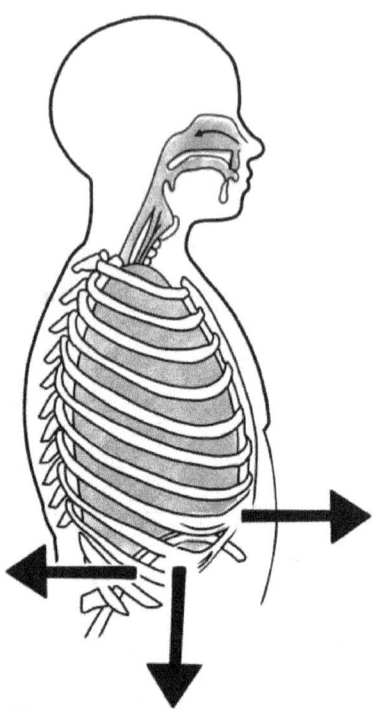

Figure 7: Optimal Breathing Pattern

There is a difference between a **Big Breath** and a **Full or Deep Breath**. Often, if I ask someone to take a big breath, they will take a big, fast breath that goes up high to the chest and may include opening the mouth. This type of breath alters the posture by shrugging the shoulders and extending the neck using accessory breathing muscles. Although this type of breath may serve a purpose, it is not an optimal diaphragmatic breath. On the other hand, a full breath will be a small, slow breath taken in through the nose that stays low in the belly. This type of breath maximizes the expansion of our lungs. Ideally, we would take full breaths at rest—not big breaths.

There are two avenues to take air to our lungs, through the nose, and through the mouth. In general, breathing in through the nose is best for our health. The nose is an important and often underappreciated organ. Outside the obvious function of smell, it is vital in optimal breathing.

James Nestor, the author of *Breath*, describes a breathing experiment that was part of his research at Stanford. The investigation included 2 phases. In Phase 1, his nose was clamped, and he was forced to breathe through his mouth for ten days. In Phase 2, he would breathe through his nose and practice breathing techniques throughout the day for the next ten days. In both phases, he would eat, sleep, and exercise normally. The researchers looked at several tests that measured pH levels, blood gasses, inflammatory markers, hormone levels, pulmonary function, heart rates, and other vital signs. The results were horrifying from a data and clinical standpoint. When he only breathed through his mouth, he developed obstructive sleep apnea, his oxygen levels dropped below 85 percent, his blood pressure was elevated, he felt lethargic, and more.[20]

Meanwhile, there are numerous benefits of nasal breathing:[21]

- Warms, humidifies, and filters the air

---

[20] Nestor, J. (2021). BREATH: THE NEW SCIENCE OF A LOST ART. PENGUIN LIFE.
[21] GRAHAM T (2012) RELIEF FROM SNORING AND SLEEP APNEA, MELBOURNE: PENGUIN GROUP (AUSTRALIA)

- Filters small and large particles through the nose hairs and mucous membranes

- Facilitates inhalation of nitric oxide, a vasodilator and bronchodilator that increases the transport of oxygen throughout the body

- Helps to prevent colds, flu, allergic reaction, and irritable coughing

- Prevents nasal dryness

- Regulates optimal airflow because of the nose's smaller, intricate passageway

- Facilitates optimal action of the diaphragm

- Promotes activity of the parasympathetic nervous system, which calms and relaxes the body, slows breathing and heart rate, and promotes digestion

- Allows for the proper position of the tongue

- Reduces the likelihood of snoring and apnea

There are times that mouth breathing is necessary and advantageous. There is not as much resistance when we breathe through our mouth because it's a bigger airway passage, so breathing in and out larger quantities of air is possible. This is important during intense physical exercise or while singing or playing a wind instrument. Mouth breathing also comes in handy when someone has difficulty breathing in through the nose, as when you have a cold. But it's not the optimal method under normal circumstances.

Breathing Faults

If a normal, healthy baby's breathing pattern is ideal, then a good comparison of a non-optimal breath pattern would be a baby with a neurological problem such as cerebral palsy or a cardiovascular problem such as a congenital heart defect. In that case, you would see:

On inspiration, the first thing to move is the chest, not the belly. The entire chest moves in an upward direction toward the head. There is less expansion of the belly and the lower rib cage out in all directions, less widening of the space between the ribs, and more elevation of the rib cage compared to the pelvis, resulting in a diagonal position of the diaphragm rather than a horizontal position.

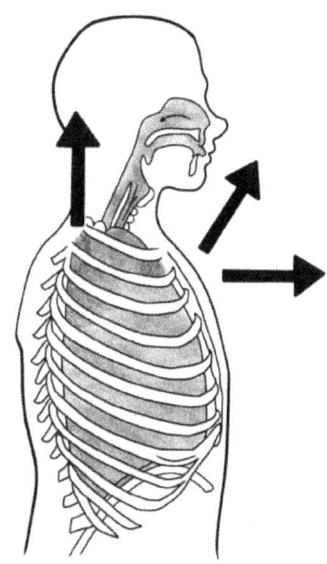

Figure 8: Non-Optimal Chest Breathing

The excursion of the diaphragm is less than complete. With the accessory breathing muscles activated, their breath may be visibly more labored and less free. Other changes in their posture include an arched back, extended head and neck, and open mouth.

An extreme medical example would be the appearance of a person who suffers from chronic obstructive pulmonary disease or emphysema. I had the terrifying experience of witnessing this with my oldest child, Jacob. He was born with a heart defect (holes in the walls of his heart), where oxygen-rich blood and oxygen-poor blood were mixed, leaving him with a lower oxygen saturation rate. He had difficulty with any activity that required physical exertion. For an infant, feeding is a high exertion activity, so his challenges were more pronounced during that time. He couldn't feed and breathe simultaneously; he would sometimes stop feeding to take a break.

After learning of his congenital heart defect just days after his birth, he was scheduled for open-heart surgery at the National Children's Hospital in Washington, DC, in 3-4 months. However, he went into respiratory distress at seven weeks of age, when his breathing worsened. I could see the manifestation of the abnormal breathing patterns above. The doctors told us to bring him to the hospital immediately for surgery.

The surgery was a complete success! The day after, my wife and I witnessed the most fantastic thing. He was able to feed while breathing simultaneously and without taking breaks. It was amazing to see how quickly he could restore a regular breathing pattern once his cardiorespiratory system was in good working order. Jacob is now 15, healthy, and has no long-standing issues from his heart condition.

Factors Inhibiting the Diaphragm's Descent

Understanding the factors inhibiting the diaphragm's optimal descent is necessary to know what we can do about them. Three things limit the inability of the diaphragm to optimally drop downward:

1. The elastic resistance of the lungs
2. The resistance of the abdominal wall
3. Postural abnormalities that create a non-parallel position of the lower rib cage as it relates to the pelvis

First, restrictive and obstructive lung diseases will affect the elasticity of the lungs. Restrictive lung diseases such as pulmonary fibrosis and pulmonary edema will limit the compliance of the lungs, causing stiffness that limits the amount of expansion. Obstructive lung diseases such as asthma, bronchitis, and emphasis cause airway obstruction, increasing the resistance so that it requires more pressure to fill a smaller volume in the lungs.

Second, anything that increases the resistance of the abdomen can limit the descent of the diaphragm. This could be due to tight-fitting clothes, belts, girdles, obesity, or excessive contraction of the abdominal muscles. All these things resist the deformation of the abdominal wall, which limits the mobility of the diaphragm downward. Ironically, excessive belly fat and six-pack abs both adversely affect your ability to breathe fully.

Third, postural abnormalities that cause lower rib cage and pelvis misalignment will minimize the diaphragm's ability to descend. The diaphragm has no space to move downward when the lower rib cage faces upward and the pelvis is tilted downward. It cannot optimally function for either its respiratory function or stabilization function. It simply has nowhere to go.

The Problem with Habitual Mouth Breathing

It is estimated that 30-50% of adults[22] and 25-57% of children[23] are mouth breathers. There are many reasons why someone may become a habitual mouth breather, including dental malocclusion, deviated nasal septum, and small nostril size, but the consequences can be considerable.

Chronic mouth breathing may contribute to:[24]

- Introduction of unfiltered, poorly dehumidified air into the lungs
- Inefficient upper chest breathing
- Chronic over-breathing
- Increased incidence of snoring and sleep apnea

---

[22] ALLEN, R. (2015). THE HEALTH BENEFITS OF NOSE BREATHING. NURSING IN GENERAL PRACTICE. HTTP://HDL.HANDLE.NET/10147/559021

[23] GREVEN, M. (2021). PREVALENCE OF MALOCCLUSION PATTERNS IN MOUTH BREATHING CHILDREN COMPARED TO NASAL BREATHING CHILDREN -A SYSTEMATIC REVIEW. THE INTERNATIONAL JOURNAL OF ORAL & MAXILLOFACIAL IMPLANTS, 7(2), 17–27.

[24] ALLEN, R. (2015). THE HEALTH BENEFITS OF NOSE BREATHING. NURSING IN GENERAL PRACTICE. HTTP://HDL.HANDLE.NET/10147/559021

- Increased probability of bad breath, gum disease, and dental decay
- Temporomandibular joint disorders (dysfunction of the jaw joint)
- Tongue thrust or poor tongue function
- Narrowing of the dental arch, jaw, and palate
- Crowded and crooked teeth
- Dental malocclusions or an open bite
- Greater potential for orthodontic corrections
- Neck, head, and jaw muscle dysfunction
- Loss of lip tone
- Speech and swallowing problems
- Trauma to soft tissues in the airways
- Enlarged tonsils and adenoids

Considering the health consequences of mouth breathing are so vast and affect people of all ages, it's unfortunate that healthcare professionals do not pay more attention to the incidence and causation of mouth breathing. It's another example of our healthcare system being more reactive than proactive. A 30–50-year female with TMJ disorders, chronic neck pain, headaches, and fatigue is told that there is nothing wrong with her because the imaging and lab studies don't show anything substantial. But the real cause may have been poor posture, malocclusion, mouth breathing, and poor breathing patterns as a child, none of which show up on an X-ray.

Like poor posture, non-optimal breathing patterns are prevalent, and not addressing them affects our physical health and well-being over the years. The actual cost of not addressing these conditions on our physical, mental, and spiritual health is unfathomable.

The breathing problems I see most commonly in my patients with chronic neck and back pain are some combination of the following:

- High resting respiratory rate
- Mouth breather
- Excessive upper chest breathing
- Reduced belly breathing or diaphragmatic breathing
- Frequent sighs or yawns
- Shallow breathing or breath-holding
- Accessory muscle overactivity
- Abdominal muscle overactivity
- Excessive belly fat
- Postural dysfunction

As adults, many of us go about our lives breathing in a non-optimal way. It affects our overall health and vitality and can lead to painful musculoskeletal conditions over time. The key is being aware of the problem and then doing something about it. In this next section, I will walk you through a self-assessment of your breathing capacity and all the signs or symptoms that may be related to a less-than-optimal breathing function.

Breathing Self-Assessment

Now that you better understand the anatomy of breathing and the difference between ideal and faulty breathing patterns, it's time to assess your breathing pattern. Before you start, take a minute to reflect on the following questions:

- How conscious are you throughout the day of your breath?
- Do you set aside time during the day to focus on breathing?
- What is the tempo or rhythm of your breath?
- Have you caught yourself shallow breathing?
- During which events throughout the day do you find your breathing rate is faster?
- Does taking a full, deep breath feel limited in any part of your body?
- How labored is your breath during certain physical activities (walking, gardening, exercise, etc.)?

The answers to these questions will give you insight into your overall awareness of your breath and the state of your subconscious breathing patterns. It will also provide insight into factors contributing to your breathing patterns during stressful events, exercise, and other active and passive times.

Next, take stock of any signs or symptoms that you may have related to poor breathing patterns. Typical symptoms can include: [25]

- Fatigue
- Frequent sighing and yawning
- Breathing discomfort
- Disturbed sleep
- Erratic heartbeats
- Feeling anxious and uptight
- Pins and needles
- Upset gut/nausea
- Clammy hands
- Chest Pains
- Shattered confidence
- Tired all the time
- Achy muscles and joints
- Dizzy spells or feeling spaced out

---

[25] CHAITOW, L., BRADLEY, D., & GILBERT, C. (2013). RECOGNIZING AND TREATING BREATHING DISORDERS: A MULTIDISCIPLINARY APPROACH (2ND ED.). CHURCHILL LIVINGSTONE.

- Irritability or hypervigilance
- Feeling of air hunger
- Chronic neck or back pain

If you suffer from several of these symptoms, your breathing pattern and ability may be compromised, contributing to your complaints.

There are also comorbidities or co-existing problems that may contribute to poor breathing patterns or dysfunctional breathing. Some of these are:

- Asthma
- Chronic Obstructive Pulmonary Disease (COPD)
- Chronic Rhinosinusitis (chronic sinus congestion)
- Chronic Pain
- Hormonal Conditions

If you have any of these conditions, you are likely to exhibit a less than optimal breathing pattern, so it will benefit you to improve your breathing function.

Nijmegen Questionnaire

This self-directed breathing questionnaire is also valuable for a self-assessment of your breathing function. The Nijmegen Questionnaire gives a broad view of symptoms associated with dysfunctional breathing patterns.[26]

This questionnaire is a specific assessment of chronic hyperventilation syndrome. A score of over 23 out of 64 suggests a positive diagnosis of hyperventilation syndrome. However, if you score below 23 but have three or more in the Often or Very Often column, this could indicate a breathing pattern disorder rather than chronic hyperventilation.

Description	Never 0	Rarely 1	Sometimes 2	Often 3	Very Often 4
Chest Pain					
Feeling Tense					
Blurred Vision					
Dizzy Spells					
Feeling Confused					

---

[26] VAN DIXHOORN, J., & FOLGERING, H. (2015). THE NIJMEGEN QUESTIONNAIRE AND DYSFUNCTIONAL BREATHING. ERJ OPEN RESEARCH, 1(1), 1–4. HTTPS://DOI.ORG/10.1183/23120541.00001-2015

Faster or Deeper Breathing						
Short of Breath						
Tight Feeling in The Chest						
Bloated Feeling in Stomach						
Tingling Fingers						
Unable to Breathe Deeply						
Stiff Fingers or Arms						
Tight Feelings around Mouth						
Cold Hands or Feet						
Palpitations						
Feeling Of Anxiety						

Are You a Mouth Breather?

It should be easy for you to answer this question. Most mouth breathers do recognize that they are. If unsure, ask your family and friends or try to notice during random moments throughout the day. If your mouth is open often and you are not naturally breathing through your nose without thinking about it, you are likely a mouth breather.

Some people know that they are because they have sinus congestion or difficulty breathing through their nose. Other signs that you may be a mouth breather include dry mouth, dry or cracked lips, bad breath, and snoring.

If you have a hard time breathing through your nose, you need to get to the root cause as to why. Seeing an ear, nose, and throat (ENT) specialist would be an excellent place to start. If it is a postural imbalance issue, seeing a physical therapist, postural specialist, or breathing specialist would be the best way to go. But wherever you go, don't put it off. Breathing through the nose is critical for a normal breathing pattern.

Breathing Self-Assessment Tests

Here's a physical self-assessment you can make of your breathing pattern in two different positions, sitting and lying on your back. This exercise will inform you about your habitual breathing pattern and whether you are limited or optimal.

Test 1: Sitting

Grab a chair and sit in front of a mirror (ideally). It's essential that you don't attempt to do any purposeful breathing or try to take a deep breath. You want to be aware of your more typical, habitual predisposition. Assess your breathing, good or bad, without trying to fix it.

1. Note whether you're breathing through your nose, mouth, or both. Are your lips touching and your mouth closed? Is it free flowing if you breathe through your nose, or does it feel constricted?

2. Place one hand on your chest and one hand on your belly. Assess which hand is moving more (the chest or the belly). If they are both moving, which moves first? If your chest is moving first or more than your belly, you are a chest breather and not breathing optimally through your diaphragm. If you try to fix this now and find that it has become exaggerated (more chest movement), that suggests there may be physical restrictions limiting optimal diaphragmatic breathing.

3. To assess your posture's role on your breathing pattern, go ahead and slouch. It's okay; I'm giving you permission. If unsure how to do this, allow your pelvis to tilt backward so your lower back rounds out and lets your spine mimic a C-curve. Now assess your breathing. Next, do the same in the opposite, overly exaggerated, over-arched lower back position. Tilt your pelvis forward so that you have maximally arched your lower back. Maintain this position and assess your breathing as you did before. How does it feel? Easy or restricted? Is your chest or belly dominant?

Test 2: Lying on Back

Lie on your back, either on a bed or on the floor. Place a pillow or small cushion under your head and knees for support. With arms by your side, let everything relax and don't create any unnecessary tension.

1. As with sitting, assess whether you're breathing through your nose or mouth. If your lips are not touching and your mouth is open, you are breathing in through your mouth. If you are breathing through your nose, is it free-flowing, or does it feel constricted? Is this the same pattern you noted in sitting, or is it different? If it is different, it may indicate some level of postural dysfunction.

2. Place one hand on your belly and one hand on your chest. Don't try to breathe in a better way, and don't try to breathe deeply. Just breathe. Assess which hand is moving first and moving more. If your chest is moving first and there is little movement of your belly hand, you are predominately a chest breather. Ideally, the initial movement is in the belly and lower rib cage. Then at the end of the expiration, there should be a slight upward movement of the rib cage and chest, but only at the end.

3. Take time to check your respiration rate. Set a timer for 1-minute and count how many rounds of breath cycles you breathe in one minute. A breath cycle comprises one inhalation

and one exhalation—average respiration rates for an adult person at rest range from **12 to 16 breaths per minute**.

Corrective Breathing Exercises

Now that you know how to identify them, it's time to get to work correcting any suboptimal breathing patterns. The best way to improve your breathing is to become more aware of it and to practice training it. A great way to start is trying these simple exercises below in the comfort of your home, sitting in your car, or while waiting in line at the store. The best part is that no one will know what you are doing. These exercises alone can bring a dramatic shift to the awareness of your breath and the role your breath plays in your overall health and, more specifically, your chronic neck and back pain.

Exercise 1: Breathing for Relaxation- Box Breathing

The first breathing exercise is the Box Breathing or Four-Square technique. The boxed breathing technique is an exercise that can promote deep breathing and reset your breath to a normal breathing rhythm. It is excellent for calming down your nervous system, inducing relaxation, and decreasing stress in your body. It can also clear your mind and help you focus if you feel agitated, stuck in your head, or distracted.

How to Do Box Breathing

Lay comfortably on your back with support under your head and legs, or sit tall in a chair or on the edge of the bed with your neck and shoulders relaxed. Place your hands on your belly to give you additional feedback and awareness of your breath.

1. Inhale slowly through your nose for a count of 4
2. Hold the breath in your lungs for a count of 4
3. Exhale slowly for a count of 4 through the nose or mouth
4. Hold the breath for a count of 4

Repeat for 5-10 cycles

Tips for Box Breathing

- Count slowly in your head
- If 4 seconds is too long, try 2 or 3 seconds
- Box breathing can be practiced anywhere
- Be cognizant of relaxing your jaw, neck, chest, and shoulder muscles throughout the exercise, as you may find that you are tensing up.

Exercise 2: Belly Breathing- Global Breathing Pattern Retraining

This belly breathing exercise will teach you how to retrain a faulty high (chest and neck) mouth-breathing pattern into a low (abdominal and lower rib cage) nose-breathing pattern. These motor control and coordination exercises are intended to teach a more regular or optimal breathing pattern. It can also help to reduce anxiety and induce relaxation.

How to Do Belly Breathing

Lie comfortably on your back with support under your head and knees. Take a deep breath and notice your current breathing pattern as you did in the self-assessment. Remember, there is a difference between taking a "big breath" and a "full breath." Don't take a big breath, which creates the opposite effect of what we are looking for here.

1. Place one hand on your belly (below the rib cage, around your belly button) and one hand on your chest.

2. Close your mouth, rest your tongue on the roof of your mouth, and ensure your teeth are not touching.

3. Breathe slowly through your nose. Feel the air move through your nose, and the pressure expand downward in your belly. The hand on the stomach should rise, while the hand on the chest should remain still.

4. Breathe out slowly through your nose or pursed lips. The belly should naturally fall toward your spine. Do not force this. You should not be creating any abdominal muscle contraction as you exhale. Let the air out effortlessly, and the belly will fall naturally. The hand on the chest should remain quiet.

Perform the exercise for 3 sets of 10 breaths. Repeat 1-3 times per day.

Tips for Belly Breathing

- Try this variation if you have difficulty allowing the belly to rise as you inhale and fall as you exhale. Place a book, small object, or weight (1-3 lbs.) on your stomach. The additional weight will give you a greater sense of feedback on the area you want to be moving.

- If you find that your back is bothering you, try resting your legs up on something (a chair, couch, or bed) to flex your hips and knees to 90 degrees. Physical therapists call this the "90-90" position. It will allow your pelvis and rib cage position to be more neutral and parallel to each other, allowing an easier breath down into the belly on your inhalation.

- Take your time. Don't force your inhalation or exhalation.

- If you find this exercise is too difficult, you may have a "reversed breath," where the habitual tendency is so strong for chest breathing that you need additional assistance or professional help in retraining your breathing pattern.

Belly Breathing Variations

Belly breathing should be practiced daily, and it may not always be convenient or feasible to practice lying on your back. Here are two other positions (sitting and lying on your stomach) that you can use to practice belly breathing. Of course, belly breathing can be practiced in standing, but it will be more difficult for most people to gain feedback in the standing position.

1. **Sitting:** Assume a good sitting posture in a chair (with or without back support) or on the edge of the bed. Place one hand on your belly and one hand on your chest. With your mouth closed, find the resting position of your jaw and tongue.

Breathe through your nose slowly, feeling the belly hand expand outward so that the chest hand remains quiet. Exhale slowly through your nose or pursed lips, allowing the belly to assume its starting position naturally. Do not contract your stomach to draw your belly inward on the exhalation.

2. **Lying on Your Stomach:** Lie on your stomach with a pillow under your pelvis if your back is uncomfortable in this position. Head can be resting on your hands with your arms overhead. Breathe in through your nose slowly and feel your belly expand against your contact with the surface below you. Exhale naturally through your nose or pursed lips. Placing a book or weight on your back can give additional feedback that may encourage belly movement.

Exercise 3: Diaphragmatic Breathing- Optimal Breathing Facilitation

Diaphragmatic breathing is all about maximizing or optimizing our natural diaphragmatic breath. The diaphragm is our primary respiratory muscle, and the more we can optimize its function and excursion, the better and deeper our natural breath will become. The diaphragm's excursion is the diaphragm's ability to move, contract, and relax to its greatest range, moving the breath further down into the belly. The result is a more significant expansion of the abdominal area and lower rib cage.

As the diaphragm contracts during inhalation, the lower rib cage expands 360 degrees around. This exercise helps to improve the excursion of the breath in the three areas that tend to lack it: the lower abdominal area, the lower side rib area, and the lower back area. If we bring awareness to these areas, we can maximize the optimal excursion of the diaphragm.

Benefits of Diaphragmatic Breathing

- Maximizes diaphragm excursion and optimal respiratory function of the diaphragm
- Relaxes tight abdominal muscles (rectus abdominis and obliques)
- Improves the function of the intercostal muscles
- Improves the mobility of the lower rib cage
- Improves the function of the internal organs by the creation of space in the abdomen
- Decreases tension of tight superficial postural muscles in the neck and back
- Relieves back pain and stiffness
- Improves breathing awareness and optimal breathing pattern
- Slows down the breathing rate
- Induces overall relaxation
- A precursor to improving the stabilization function of the diaphragm

How to Do Diaphragmatic Breathing

1. Lie comfortably on your back with your feet flat, knees bent, and support under your head.

2. Close your mouth, rest your tongue on the roof of your mouth, and ensure your teeth are not touching.

3. **Lower Abdominal Focus**: Place the fingertips of both hands between the belly button and the pubic bone (hard bone above your genital area). Breathe in slowly through your nose. Feel the movement with your fingers in the lower abdominal region. Try to expand this movement out into your fingertips during the inhalation. Don't force it, but try to improve it by gently pushing it out into your fingertips as you breathe in. Breathe out slowly through your nose or pursed lips. You can also think about breathing low into your pelvis area to help facilitate breathing into the lower abdominal region.

    Repeat for 10 breaths.

4. **Lower Side Rib Focus**: Place the palms of both hands to the side of your lower ribs on each side (your elbows will be pointing out to the sides). If you don't have the mobility in your arms or it bothers your shoulder to place your hands in this position, instead put your elbows snug to your body so that your elbows are contacting your lower side ribs. Breathe in slowly through your nose. Feel the movement with your palms (or elbows) in the lower side ribs. Try to expand this movement out during the inhalation. Don't force it, but try to improve it

by gently pushing it out into your palms as you breathe in. Breathe out slowly through your nose or pursed lips. Depending on your posture and inherent muscle imbalances, there may not be much movement here.

Repeat for 10 breaths.

5. **Lower Back Focus**: Place the palms of both hands to the side of your lower ribs on each side (as you did for the side ribs), but now also be sure that your thumbs are resting in the space between the last rib and the pelvis in the backside area of your lower back. It should feel like a slight indentation (crater) that your thumbs will naturally fall into. Breathe in slowly through your nose. Feel the movement with your thumbs in the lower back area. Try to expand this movement out during the inhalation. Don't force it, but try to improve it by gently pushing out into your thumbs as you breathe in. Think about breathing into your back or the surface you are lying on. Breathe out slowly through your nose or pursed lips. Depending on your posture and inherent muscle imbalances, there may not be much movement here.

Repeat for 10 breaths.

Perform the exercise for 10 breaths in each position and repeat 1-3 times per day.

Tips for Diaphragmatic Breathing

- You are still belly breathing with all three exercise variations, but you are focusing each set on the awareness and the ability to breathe into different areas.

- If you find it difficult to breathe into any of the three areas discussed above, try changing your starting positions. Instead of lying on your back with your feet flat and knees bent, try lying in the 90-90 position so that your legs are resting on a chair, couch, or bed, allowing your hips and knees to be in a 90-degree position. This will assist in a more optimal lower rib cage and pelvis alignment, allowing the diaphragm to descend into the stomach more easily.

- If you find that you are having difficulty breathing into the lower abdominal area, try this variation. Place a small object or weight (1-3 lbs.) on your lower abdominal area between the belly button and pubic bone. The additional weight will give you a greater sense of feedback in the area you want to be moving.

- If you have difficulty breathing into the lower side ribs, try wrapping a band or belt around your lower rib cage. It should be snug but not so tight to not allow rib movement. Now breathe into the band or belt as you inhale, gently pushing out sideways against the feedback of the band or belt.

- If you have difficulty breathing into the lower back ribs, try using a tennis ball or rolled-up socks to give feedback. Place a small ball or rolled-up socks under the lower back ribs and above the pelvis on each side between your rib cage and the floor. With your lower ribs slightly elevated away from the floor, the ball or sock should fit nicely into this space. Breathe into the ball or sock as you breathe in.

- Take your time. Don't force your inhalation. Make it slow and full. Don't force the exhalation. Let the belly retract naturally without any abdominal muscle contraction.

- If you still find this exercise very difficult, you may have postural dysfunction (e.g., tight muscles or stiff rib cage/spine) that is significant enough to prohibit movement in these areas. In that case, you should seek the professional help of a physical therapist, massage therapist, chiropractor, or personal trainer to work on these physical limitations first.

Diaphragmatic Breathing Variations

Diaphragmatic breathing should be practiced daily. It is preferable to practice while lying on your back, but it can also be practiced on your stomach, side, or sitting. You will still breathe into the three different areas for 10 breaths using your hands or other forms of feedback to facilitate the awareness and movement of these areas.

1. **Lying on Your Stomach:** Lie on your stomach with a pillow under your pelvis if your back is uncomfortable in this position. Head can be resting on your hands with your arms overhead. Breathe through your nose slowly and feel the expansion into your lower abdominal area, side ribs, and lower back.

2. **Lying on Your Side:** Lie on your side with a pillow under your head, and a pillow between your legs, hips, and knees flexed to 90 degrees. Feel the expansion of movement into the lower abdominals, lower side ribs, and lower back ribs using your hands and fingertips for feedback on the inhalation.

3. **Sitting:** Assume a good sitting posture in a chair (with or without back support) or on the edge of the bed. As you slowly breathe in, feel the expansion of movement into the lower abdominals, lower side ribs, and lower back ribs using your hands and fingertips. This is an excellent position to practice the sideways expansion using a band or belt around your lower ribs.

Exercise 4: Prolonged Exhalation Breathing: Optimal Volume & Metabolic Balance

If you want to improve your inhalation, one way is to focus on improving your exhalation. It sounds counterintuitive, but it's true. Most people try to take a bigger inhalation to improve their breathing, thinking it will get more oxygen into their system. If done to excess or repeated quickly, this focus on bigger, faster inhalations can lead to hyperventilation and a deficiency of carbon dioxide in the bloodstream and body (hypocapnia). What they should be doing is the opposite.

To re-establish the metabolic balance of oxygen and carbon dioxide in your bloodstream, you need to reduce breath volume and slow the breath down. The best way to do that is to prolong your exhalation.

Benefits of Prolonged Exhalation Breathing

- Increases carbon dioxide levels in the blood
- Reduces hyperinflation of the lungs
- Makes more efficient use of oxygen
- Stimulates the parasympathetic nervous system response (decreases heart rate and dilates blood vessels)
- Decreases muscle tension
- Decreases heart-rate variability
- Induces relaxation and calming effect

How to Do Prolonged Exhalation Breathing

1. Lie comfortably on your back with your feet flat, knees bent, and support under your head.
2. Close your mouth, rest your tongue on the roof of your mouth, and ensure your teeth are not touching.
3. Breathe in for 4 seconds
4. Pause for 2 seconds before beginning your exhalation
5. Breathe out slowly through pursed lips for 8 seconds
6. Pause for 2 seconds before beginning your inhalation
7. Repeat for 10 cycles. Work up to doing this for 10 minutes per day

Tips for Prolonged Exhalation Breathing

- If 4 seconds in and 8 seconds out is too long, or if you are really struggling to catch your breath, decrease the time. Stick to a 1:2 ratio, so 3 seconds in and 6 seconds out or 2 seconds in and 4 seconds out.

- This will initially seem uncomfortable, but it will become easier with practice.

- As you get better, you can experiment with breathing out until you have nothing left to breathe out and work on prolonged holds at the maximum exhalation for 6-8 seconds.

- Practice daily for maximum effect.

- This is one of the most beneficial exercises you can do to restore your optimal breath.

Conclusion

I hope you have come to appreciate the importance of optimal breathing as it relates to your overall health and wellbeing. Try out these four simple breathing techniques and exercises. If you stick with it, you will not be disappointed. There is no doubt you will experience positive short-term effects and even long-term effects. Improving your breathing ability is a great starting point in addressing your chronic neck and lower back pain, and it may be the most important thing you can do to improve your overall physical, emotional, and spiritual health.

CHAPTER 7

Activating the Core

"Core stabilization is a prerequisite of any locomotion function. Abnormal stabilization compromises the quality of any dynamic movement."

Pavel Kolář, PT, PHD

Our Core Inner Stability

When treating someone with a spinal condition in the clinic, especially a chronic one, I always start with restoring an optimal breathing pattern. Why? Other than the numerous health benefits of improving your breath, when it comes to your core or postural stability, if you can't breathe into an area, then you can't stabilize that area.

The optimization of the respiratory function of the diaphragm allows us to optimize the stabilization function of the diaphragm. The intra-abdominal pressure is the foundation of our postural stability. The intra-abdominal pressure protects and maintains our spine health. And the intra-abdominal pressure can optimize our ability to move.

This chapter is about this intra-abdominal pressure, which is the basis of our deep spinal stability and, therefore, our postural stability. It will discuss the importance of intra-abdominal pressure related to our spine health and movement function, what creates this abdominal pressure, and how and why it's at the root of most chronic neck and back pain. This will allow you to become more aware of this pressure and learn exercises to improve upon creating and maintaining it.

We will be talking about babies again because this method is exactly what babies must do in the first year of life to be able to start to move and to be able to progress through the developmental stages that result in their ability to upright themselves up against gravity, to crawl, to stand, and to walk, all without being taught or trained by anyone. They do it naturally, and so can you.

If you improve your spinal stability, core stability, and postural stability, you will help your chronic neck and back condition. After all, the most common cause of neck and back pain is overloading the spine, and the spine becomes overloaded over time due to the incorrect function or the incapacity of the spinal stabilization muscle system to counteract the load.

Almost every neck and back condition can be attributed to this, including disc herniations, spinal stenosis, spondylolisthesis, degenerative disc disease, spinal facet joint arthritis, radiculopathy (nerve impingement), sciatica, muscle spasm, and guarding. They are all manifestations of overloading of the spine over time and the inability of the deep spinal stability system to counteract or stabilize the load.

A disc herniation results from the outer layer of the disc weakening and tearing, causing bulges and herniations. The reason it weakens and ultimately tears are excessive load forces over time. Degenerative disc disease results from compressive forces that cause the discs to break down and lose disc height over time. Why do they break down and lose height over time? Overload. Spondylolisthesis is the slippage of one vertebra over another, potentially causing some spinal instability because of the load on the spine. Same with spinal facet joint arthritis, where compressive loads on the spinal joints start a process of degeneration over time. Nerve impingement, sciatica, muscle spasms, and guarding are all secondary consequences of this overload.

There's a reason these spinal conditions tend to be found in consistent places along the spine, in the junctions between the head and the neck, the lower neck and the upper back, the mid-back and the upper lower back, the lower back and the tailbone (the sacrum), and the tailbone and the pelvis (sacroiliac joint). They are all in areas of the spine that tend to have hypermobility issues with biomechanical overload.

These spinal medical diagnoses are not the problem. They are the result of the problem. It's not arthritis or nerve impingement that is the problem. They are the secondary consequences of an overloaded spine and the inadequate ability of the spinal stabilization system to counteract this load. These diagnoses may cause acute or recurrent pain, whether chemical inflammatory pain, mechanical impingement pain, or neuropathic pain, but relieving the symptoms of this pain will not solve the problem. They may be the smoke, but they are not what caused the fire.

All of us have these conditions at some point in life, as any X-ray or MRI will show, but we are not always in pain. It is only when we have an imbalance between the load placed on our bodies and our physical capacity to handle the load that the symptoms will manifest themselves. This can be due to an acute injury/trauma or chronic overloading.

What creates a load on our spine? Gravity, prolonged improper posturing, and poor-quality movement patterns. All these factors influence our bodies, our structure, and our tissues. Our capacity to accept these loads day in and day out will be the difference.

For example, if you have poor physical capacity (i.e., poor posture, genetic hypermobility, scoliosis) and the load is low or moderate, this will likely mean no symptoms or pain. Poor capacity with a medium to high load (running, exercise, sitting for 8 hours a day) equals an imbalance that will manifest as back pain or neck pain at some point, whether transient or consistent.

The inverse is also true. Someone with decent physical capacity and a low or moderate load will usually be asymptomatic (despite what their x-ray or MRI might say). However, even someone with good capacity (i.e., a young person, fit adult, athlete) can experience symptoms with a high load over time (excessive workouts, excessive weight training, excessive running mileage, etc.).

The balanced activation of the spinal stability muscles allows for loading the spine's parts more symmetrically, reducing overload. Poor quality of activation of this system results in overloading certain aspects of our spine, leading to possible arthritic changes, disc herniations, and nerve compression.

To prevent potential pain and injury, you have two basic options: decrease your load or improve your capacity. This book is about improving your capacity to accept and counteract the load, not in a compensatory way, but in a healthy way from the inside out.

How do you improve the internal capacity to correct and counter the overload and prevent neck and back pain? The answer is enhancing the activity and coordination of your spinal stabilization muscle system, which comprises abdominal muscles, the diaphragm, the pelvic floor, and back muscles. This includes improving your breathing patterns.

This chapter will teach you the basic principles of the correct activation of the spinal or trunk stability system and provide some individual exercises for you to try on your own. Much of this may counter what you have heard from others or what you have come to understand about the core.

You won't hear "engage your core," "tighten your stomach," "draw your belly button in," "hollow your belly," or "suck in your belly." Those engage the superficial muscles, which is precisely the wrong thing to do.

You will hear "breath low," "push out," "create pressure," "breathe and brace," "breathe and pressurize," and "maintain the pressure as you breathe." This is how you get stronger from the inside out.

Anatomy & Function

The core is the set of muscles around our trunk that make up the basis of our spinal and postural stability. Although people often talk about "activating" or "engaging" the core, it is always active, even at rest, because its primary function is to stabilize the spine and create a foundation from which our extremities can move. And that's what the body is ultimately meant to do—move.

We discussed the anatomy of the spine at the start of Chapter 5 on posture, but let's briefly review it here for context. Our spinal column comprises a series of vertebrae, spinal discs, ligaments, and soft tissue (muscles and fascia). The vertebrae are connected via the discs and ligaments, which give the spinal segments some passive stability. This baseline passive stability is essential and can be compromised by macrotrauma injuries such as car accidents and falls or by microtrauma forces acting on the spine from daily activities such as sitting, bending, and lifting. The spinal column has 26 bones, consisting of the cervical spine (C1-7), thoracic spine (T1-12), lumbar spine (L1-5), sacrum (fused vertebrae), and coccyx (tailbone).

A spinal segment or spinal joint comprises the vertebrae above, the disc in between, and the vertebrae below. Ligaments attach to them, and the connections between the vertebrae are known as the uncinate and facet joints. The joints between the spine and the ribs allow the spine to be a mobile structure capable of forward bending, backward bending, side bending, and rotating. The combination of all these little joints moving individually allows the spine to move as a whole. Thus, all body movements, big or small, result in spine movement.

The structure we have described thus far is mobile but relatively weak. The bones are strong, but the connections between them are fragile. They can only withstand a small amount of stress (less than 10 kilograms) before being injured. They wouldn't be able to support our body weight on their own. Instead, they rely on the muscular system.

The spinal muscular system is made up of stabilizers and movers. The stabilizing muscles are short, small muscles that lie close to the spine structure spanning 1 to 3 vertebrae. The purpose of these muscles is to stabilize the spinal segments. They control the spine and prevent excessive motion. The movement muscles are longer and thicker muscles that lie further from the spine structure. These muscles create more significant gross movements of the spine, such as bending and twisting. The superficial muscles tend to have a power-generating function, while the deeper muscles tend to have control and stability functions.

To understand what makes up a healthy, stable spine, it helps to think of three layers of spinal muscle anatomy: deep, middle, and superficial.

The three deep muscles of the back include the semispinalis, multifidus, and rotatores. These short, small muscles stabilize the vertebral column and play a role in proprioception. These muscles help with intricate movements, control of spinal vertebrae, and postural stability.

The middle layers of muscles include the quadratus lumborum in the back and psoas in the front. In the neck, it consists of the scalenus, splenius capitis, and splenius cervicis. These muscles are larger and longer than the deeper muscles, spanning 5-7 segments. Some of these muscles have a primary movement function, and some primarily have stabilization functions. Two of these muscles strongly contribute to the adaptive guarding or stabilization function—the quadratus lumborum and psoas muscles in the back.

The middle layer muscles also connect different areas of the body. The quadratus lumborum connects the lower ribs to the pelvis, the spine to the pelvis, and the lower ribs to the spine. The psoas connects the spine to the pelvis. The scalene connects the upper rib cage to the neck. The splenius capitis connects the lower neck to the head. The splenius cervicis connects the lower neck to the outside of the upper neck. This means they can be prone to compensations and imbalances. For instance, the quadratus lumborum and psoas tend to compensate and guard in longstanding chronic neck and back conditions, usually on one side more than the other. It's hard to restore optimal mobility and stability unless these muscles are adequately addressed and normalized in length and tone.

The superficial layer of muscles includes the superficial extensors in the back (longissimus, iliocostalis, and spinalis), the rectus abdominis in the front, and the oblique abdominals (internal and external obliques). These are long, superficial muscles that flex, extend, side bend, and rotate the spine and rib cage, so they tend to become tight, full of trigger points, and tender to the touch. These muscles are often the source of pain, and alleviating trigger points in these muscles is often necessary.

The other muscles that make our spinal stability are the diaphragm above, the pelvic floor below, the deepest abdominal muscle (transverse abdominis) in the front, and the deepest back muscles (multifidi) in the back. The coactivation of these muscles creates the intra-abdominal pressure that pushes back against the spine, gives support, and activates other deep stabilizing muscles from the spine to the head.

If you want to stabilize your spine, it isn't done by strengthening the superficial muscles of your neck and back. It is done by creating and controlling intra-abdominal pressure.

Sit-ups and back extensions are not the way to strengthen your back or core. If anything, you may be compounding your back problems. It is better not to think of this system as something that needs strengthening. Rather than strength, what you need most is awareness, coordination, and control.

Ideal Postural Stability

Improving postural stability is the best way to address most of your chronic low back and neck problems. Why? Because postural stabilization is the active muscle stability required to maintain body segments against gravity and external forces. These forces overload and break down parts of our spine and joints. Improving postural stability will help your body withstand these forces and minimize the overloading that leads to wear and tear.

Postural stabilization is necessary for static positions such as prolonged sitting and standing, and all dynamic movement. Any movement of your arms, legs, or head, whether lifting your arm to reach for something, lifting your leg to take a step, or getting up out of bed, requires a certain amount of postural stability before that movement can occur. Many scientific studies have shown that muscle activity in postural muscles occurs before and during movement. But we don't need to study this in a lab to understand it. We can see it in how babies move in the first year of their life.

By the third month, as a baby's central nervous system develops, its ability to coordinate and control intra-abdominal pressure improves. The baby begins to coordinate all the diaphragm functions of breathing, stability, and sphincter control. The control of the intra-abdominal pressure gives the spinal stability to elongate and lift the spine against gravity and gives the postural stability necessary to begin to move.

A baby on its back at five months of age can control intra-abdominal pressure to the degree that it can raise its head, arms, and legs up against the resistance of gravity. The intra-abdominal pressure creates stability of the spine. Spinal stability is the foundation for synergistic muscle activities that allow the distal muscles to move limbs. It all starts with the stability of the spine and postural stability. As the baby further improves its ability to stabilize on their back and lift their head and limbs, they start to control that stability for turning and rolling on to their side, then up on their elbows, then up on their hands, then transferring onto their hands and knees, and so on until they can fully walk and move.

Stability comes before mobility. The stability gained from the intra-abdominal pressure acting on the spine feeds into the stability of other parts of our bodies, mainly our shoulder and hip girdle, which allows for the movement of the limbs.

A baby on hands and knees at six months old is a perfect example. This position is called the "quadruped" position. Stability in this position is a prerequisite for crawling. The baby has made it to its hands and knees and is now learning to control the intra-abdominal pressure in this position. But it's not the core or the intra-abdominal pressure on its own that allows the baby to maintain this position. Stability within the shoulder girdle and the hip girdle is also necessary.

The baby rocks back and forth and side to side, further challenging its ability to stabilize itself and learning to load its hands and knees. The baby is driven to move. The ability to crawl by bringing one arm forward and the opposite knee ahead requires learning how to stabilize the opposing limbs first. This is called the support function. To lift its right hand to bring it forward in front of her, it must stabilize the left hand on the ground with the synergistic series of muscle activity stabilizing the left shoulder girdle. In conjunction with the spinal/postural stability that has already been established, the shoulder girdle stability of the left arm gives the baby the ability to unweight its right arm to move it forward. This is called the movement function.

The same is true in the lower body for a baby to bring its knee forward to crawl. It must stabilize on the opposite knee through the hip girdle to move the leg forward. Eventually, it improves its postural stability to unweight the opposite arm and opposite leg forward simultaneously to be able to crawl. This coordinated effort to stabilize then move happens in every single developmental position. The baby's ability to practice and improve this ability allows for the developmental progression from rolling to crawling, standing, and walking.

The stages of different positions and movements a baby goes through in the first year of life are a continuous example of how and why stability precedes mobility. At every step, the support function precedes the movement function.

For another illustration, imagine a post embedded into the ground with a rope attached to the top. If the post is stable in the ground, pulling on the rope, once you take up the slack, will create maximal tension in the rope, making it unable to move any farther. Now imagine the post is embedded loosely in the ground. In this case, when you pull on the rope, the post will give and move a little.

The post represents your spine, and the rope represents a muscle. Every muscle has attachments to one or more bones called the origin and insertion. So, any lengthening or contraction of a muscle will influence the bones or joints they are attached to, just as pulling on the rope affects the post. If the origin bone is not stable when that muscle contracts or lengthens, its ability to create tension in a muscle will be determined by the sturdiness of the bone it is attached to. Any muscle contraction will be less than ideal if the bone is not stable. Continuous shortening and lengthening will tug on that unstable attachment, making it more unstable, like the post wiggling loose in the ground.

A clinical example of this is in the primary hip flexor muscle, the iliopsoas. This muscle attaches from the front of the lower spine to the front of the thigh bone. You contract your iliopsoas when you actively pull your knee toward your chest while standing. This movement is called hip flexion. But if you are standing still and your iliopsoas are contracted, it pulls in the reverse direction, causing your lower spine to go into relative extension or a forward pelvic tilt.

In the first instance, the spine is the post, and the hip flexor is the rope so that the spine will determine the hip flexors' coordination and strength. If that spinal origin is not fixed and stable, the hip flexor will not be as coordinated or strong, and compensations by other muscles and parts of the body will occur. Over time, an imbalance between the load and the capacity would cause hip flexor tendonitis, active trigger points in the muscle with pain or muscle dysfunction, limited hip extension mobility due to hip flexor tightness, or possible sacroiliac joint dysfunction.

On the other hand, if you are standing and your foot is fixed to the ground, any overactivity or increased tension of the hip flexors will pull on the point of attachment to the spine, pulling it forward and causing extension forces on the spine. This could manifest into signs and symptoms of spinal stenosis, spondylolisthesis, compression of the lumbar spine, or sacroiliac joint dysfunction.

You can see these constantly in sports and physical performance. The martial artist gets the power and speed of their punch from their core, not their arm strength. The golfer generates the power of his golf swing from the stability of his core and the reaction forces from the ground, not from his arms. The same is true for the baseball player hitting or throwing a baseball. It's not the arm strength; it's the ability of the body to create stability where forces can be generated powerfully and efficiently. The same is true for a soccer player kicking a ball. It's not the leg strength; the postural stability and single-leg stability of the opposite leg create the foundation for the soccer player to swing the kicking leg effectively, efficiently, and effortlessly, allowing for the big kick. Most athletes know this instinctively. This is why pitchers don't usually have the most muscular arms, and the soccer player who can kick the farthest doesn't have the big, bulging legs of a bodybuilder.

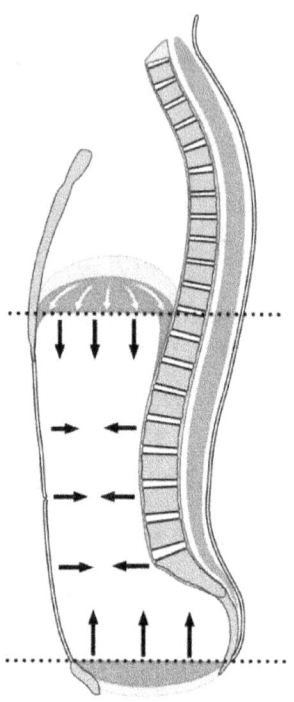

Figure 9: Optimal Postural Stability

Pictures published with permission from Rehabilitation Prague School www.rehabps.com

This spinal and postural stability starts with the creation of intra-abdominal pressure. The intra-abdominal pressure is created by the coactivation of the diaphragm above, the pelvic floor below, the deep transverse abdominis muscle in the front, and the deep multifidi back muscles (see Figure 9). Perhaps the most critical aspect of this system is the diaphragm muscle. Without its role in creating downward pressure, optimal intra-abdominal pressure and stability wouldn't be possible. This is the stabilization function of the diaphragm, the ability to stay down, when necessary, to remain contracted and engaged when activities require a certain amount of postural stability. There are also times when the diaphragm kicks in automatically, such as while coughing, sneezing, swallowing, laughing, or crying.

The diaphragm also has additional visceral and sphincter functions that are not often recognized. Dysfunction of the diaphragm can contribute to common conditions such as constipation and gastroesophageal reflux disease (GERD). Many people suffer from these common conditions, but rarely do I ever hear someone mention the role of improving diaphragmatic function in these conditions. More commonly, the non-functional medical approach has addressed these problems through medication.

Non-Ideal Postural Stability

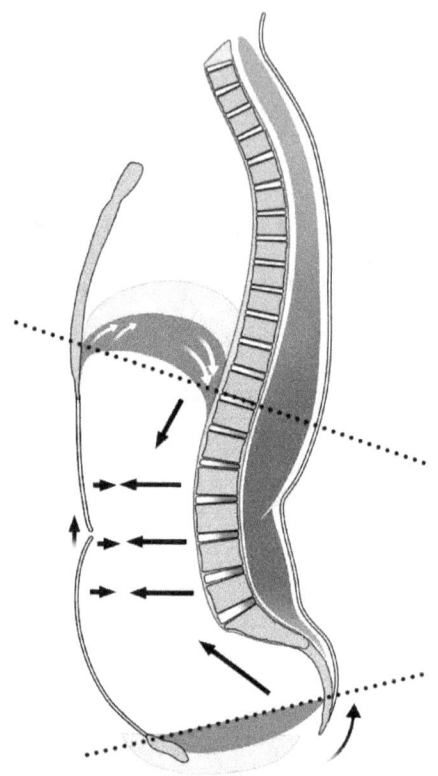

Figure 10: Non-Optimal Postural Stability

Pictures published with permission from Rehabilitation Prague School www.rehabps.com

The body's musculoskeletal and nervous systems have an incredible ability to adapt over time. As adolescents and adults, we don't have to stabilize perfectly to move, walk, run, or jump. We adjust and compensate. Adaptation is inevitable.

However, the degree to which we compensate and the amount of load placed on us determine whether or not that adaptation damages our musculoskeletal system. It is not always clear cut, but if our postural and spinal stability system is less than ideal, we risk developing musculoskeletal symptoms over time. This is true of every stage of life.

With dysfunctional spinal and postural stability, our ability to create optimal intra-abdominal pressure is compromised. In Figure 10, you see that the lower rib cage is elevated so that the diaphragm is tilted upward, oriented diagonally instead of horizontally. You also see that the pelvis is tilted downward, changing the angle of the pelvis and the orientation of the pelvic floor. With this anatomical alignment, the diaphragm cannot descend optimally, and the pelvic floor can not counteract the downward pressure of the diaphragm because they don't sit parallel to one another. You also see the overactivity of the superficial abdominal and back muscles. As a result, intra-abdominal pressure is not as efficient. The body will still attempt to stabilize and engage when our daily activities require postural stability, but it will be inefficient and result in overactivity of the superficial muscles, overloading compression of the spinal structures, and creating a less than stable basis for movement.

While adolescents and adults don't have to stabilize perfectly to move—babies do. If they don't stabilize, they aren't going anywhere. But if their development is affected by a condition or is delayed, compensations can start to set in. For example, a baby who has suffered a neurological deficit or disorder, such as cerebral palsy, will demonstrate the characteristics of non-ideal postural stability. Their back will arch with lower ribs flared outward. Their chest will be high, and their neck will be hyperextended with poor neck and head control. Their breathing will be less than ideal and high in their chest. Their superficial neck and shoulder muscles, abdominal muscles, and back muscles will be hyperactive. The movements of limbs will lack smoothness and control.

When on their stomach, this baby will display hyperactivity of their superficial back muscles, hyperextension of their neck and shrugging of the shoulders, and hyperactivity of their buttock and hamstring muscles. All these impairments are due to less-than-optimal postural spinal stability, affecting the quality of movement as they develop in the first year of life.

A baby doesn't necessarily need a neurological disorder to display such impairments. A baby may demonstrate early signs of poor coordination and motor difficulties, commonly known as Developmental Coordination Disorder (DCD). Children with DCD may be delayed in early developmental milestones such as crawling, standing, and walking. They may have difficulty with everyday physical activities as they age, from riding a bike to jumping to kicking a ball. Often these kids are described as clumsy or accident-prone, but the problems usually stem from unaddressed motor development problems in the first year of life. Parents of these kids have been told that their child will grow out of it, and sometimes that is true. Still, these kids would be much better off physically if they had been appropriately assessed for poor postural stability early in their development.

As children become more active in physical activities and sports, any impairments of coordination and movement can manifest as problems. In my twenty-plus years of practice, I have consistently been amazed by the high number of kids who suffer injuries and are in pain. I'll never forget the first time one of my patients told me her 12-year-old daughter was also suffering from persistent back pain. Kids aren't supposed to be complaining of back pain.

I believe this growing incidence of pain in kids is due to an imbalance between the load placed on our kids and their capacity to withstand these loads. The load comes in the form of heavy backpacks, prolonged sitting postures, and earlier onset of computer use. And for those involved in youth sports, the load is clearly due to longer and more frequent practices and games along with the focus on a specific sport year-round without varying their sports activities throughout the year.

The same is true in young and middle-aged adults, except it is worse. More persistent and recalcitrant because adults have lived more years with imbalances and compensations. More years of wear and tear. More years of shearing and compressive forces. More years of muscle overloading and overactivity. More years of fascial tightness. More years of injuries and traumas.

It sounds awful, but it doesn't have to be, and it doesn't have to equal symptoms. The mere presence of an impairment (muscle imbalances, poor posture, poor stability) doesn't necessarily equal pain. Pain will result either from an acute injury or from overload, excessive stress, or excessive strain over time that the neuromusculoskeletal system cannot withstand. Tendonitis, bursitis, disc herniations, nerve impingements, joint inflammation, painful trigger points, etc. These are the musculoskeletal implications of a system that cannot meet its demands.

In younger or middle-aged adults, these problems typically will show themselves after a person decides to start exercising again or increase the frequency and intensity of an existing exercise program. Folks starting to exercise after the new year is a perfect example.

Here's a typical presentation. A 40-year-old woman decides to get back in shape after the new year. She joins a gym and starts an exercise routine that involves cardio and lifting weights using machines and dumbbells. It's been years since she exercised regularly, and she is not in the same physical condition as in her twenties. A month after she started exercising, she began to have neck pain. She says she felt like her neck got tweaked or kinked. Now she has neck pain after every workout, she is waking up with neck pain, and she has lost mobility in her neck, making it difficult to turn her head while driving. She tries taking care of it herself and modifies her exercises by lessening the weight, but the problem continues. This person will likely be diagnosed with a muscle strain. She will have painful, tight muscles in her neck with limited spinal joint mobility. This person typically responds very quickly to dry needling and manual therapy, experiencing significantly less pain and improved mobility within a few sessions.

However, while the trigger points and the spinal restrictions may have been the cause of the pain and limited mobility, what caused them to be problematic is poor postural spinal stability. That lack of stability contributes to her performing exercises with poor quality and compensation, overusing her superficial neck muscles, which causes an acute neck muscle spasm and inflammation of the small joints of the spine.

The possible reasons for the poor postural spinal stability are numerous. It may be due to past injuries, trauma, pregnancy, or a genetic predisposition to hypermobility. Everyone is different, and each of us has a unique history, physical make-up, genetic predisposition, past injuries and traumas, and life experiences that uniquely affect our bodies.

Now, look at a 75-year-old man with low back pain and difficulty with prolonged standing and walking. If he stands or walks for 15 minutes, low back pain and pain down both legs start, after which he must sit to relieve his symptoms. This person has a long-standing history of low back pain and was a manual laborer. His doctor has told him that he has spinal stenosis (narrowing the space where the nerves come out of the spine), and the MRI confirms the diagnosis.

His symptom presentation also confirms the diagnosis. Those with spinal stenosis tend not to tolerate extension-type physical activities such as prolonged standing and walking because standing erect causes more spine extension, decreasing the space where the nerve roots exit the spine. Various things can be done in therapy to address this problem. Restoring flexion mobility of the lower back and improving extension of the hips will help because those imbalances contribute to the excessive extension of the lower spine that can cause and aggravate the symptoms.

But that is not enough. The postural spinal stability must be addressed for long-term relief. The intra-abdominal pressure that creates optimal postural spinal stability pushes back against the front of the spine, supporting it and giving it elongation. The result is an improved capacity to maintain upright, erect postures with less compression and impingement of the nerves in the lumbar spine. Achieving this requires active correction by improving the stability system's awareness, endurance, and robustness. Otherwise, his lower spine will never be stable enough to support him and create space in his lower back.

When I point out the deficiencies of the stability system to my patients, they get it on a deeper level. They just wish they would have learned about all this sooner. Yet they often feel pessimistic about their underlying instability, believing it somehow reflects poorly on them and their ability to function optimally over the years.

I try to get my patients to understand that their awareness of the problem will ultimately be their solution. And while it is true that we all could have benefited from better training and education on how to move correctly when we were younger, we can still set ourselves up for a better future regarding our physical health. I tell my patients not to feel bad about any deficiencies and impairments; it means their body has compensated well over the years. It did what was necessary to deal with its demands. This is normal. Now that they understand how it relates to their problem, they can finally do something to fix it permanently without the use of medication, injections, and surgery.

Core Stability Self-Assessment

Now that you understand the functional anatomy of postural stability, optimal postural stability, and non-ideal postural stability, it's time to assess yourself. First, take a moment to reflect on the following questions:

- How conscious are you throughout the day of your core or postural stability?

- How much time do you set aside during the day to focus on your core or postural stability?

- What percentage of your exercise routine is dedicated to improving your core or postural stability?

- How would you rate your ability to properly engage your core and postural stability based on what you now know?

- How aware are you of your core and postural stability throughout an exercise routine?

- How aware are you of your core and postural stability throughout prolonged positions (sitting, standing, driving)?

- How aware are you of your core and postural stability throughout daily physical activities (walking, lifting, carrying, gardening, etc.)?

It is also helpful to understand the signs or symptoms you may have related to spinal instability. You will find typical signs and symptoms of instability in this questionnaire, adapted from the Clinimetric Testing of the Lumbar Spine Instability Questionnaire.[27] The questionnaire was aimed initially toward the lower back. Still, it applies to neck instability as well.

Lumbar Spine Instability Questionnaire

Answer "Yes" or "No" to the following questions regarding your back or neck condition.

1. I feel like my back/neck is going to "give way" or "give out" on me
2. I feel the need to frequently pop my back/neck
3. I have frequent bouts or episodes of symptoms
4. In the past, my back/neck catches or locks when I twist or bend my spine

---

[27] Saragiotto, B. T., Maher, C. G., New, C. H., Catley, M., Hancock, M. J., Cook, C. E., & Hodges, P. W. (2018). Clinimetric Testing of the Lumbar Spine Instability Questionnaire. The Journal of orthopaedic and sports physical therapy, 48(12), 915–922. https://doi.org/10.2519/jospt.2018.7866

5. I experience pain when I change positions (e.g., sit-to-stand or stand-to-sit)

6. When I bend forward it hurts, but returning to standing is usually worse

7. My pain increases with quick, unexpected, or mild movements

8. I have difficulty sitting without a back support (such as a chair) and feel better with a supportive backrest

9. My pain is usually worse with prolonged or static positions

10. It seems like my condition is getting worse over time (e.g., shorter intervals between bouts)

11. I have had this problem a long time

12. I get temporary pain relief with a back/neck brace or corset

13. I have many occasions when I get muscle spasms in the back/neck

14. I am sometimes fearful to move because of my pain

15. I have had a back/neck injury or trauma in the past

Give yourself **1 point** for the questions you answered **Yes and add up your total score**. A higher score indicates a greater probability of a spinal instability subset of chronic back or neck pain. If you suffer from several of these signs and symptoms, the underlying root cause of your problem is probably a lack of deep spinal or postural stability contributing to the spinal disc, joint, nerve, and muscle dysfunction.

Other Contributing Comorbidities

Also, comorbidities or co-existing problems may affect or be affected by non-optimal spinal stability. Some of these include:

- Scoliosis
- Spondylolisthesis (slippage of one vertebra over another)
- Thoracic Hyperkyphosis (excessive curvature of the mid-back)
- Lumbar Hyperlordosis (excessive curvature of the lower back)
- Trauma affecting the spine (car accidents, falls, compression fractures, head trauma, etc.)
- Systemic hypermobility and Ehlers Danlos Syndrome
- Post-Partum
- Childhood development issues

If you have any of these conditions, you are likely to exhibit less than optimal spinal stability, and it would benefit you to improve your postural stability function.

Lower Back Self-Assessment Tests

A few self-assessment tests you can do at home may indicate whether you have a spinal instability problem. I will give a couple for your back and your neck. Please take care in these movements and do not do them if you know or suspect it may aggravate your back or neck symptoms. If in doubt, don't do them and seek the evaluation of a physical therapist who can administer and assess these tests and more with minimal risk of aggravation.

Test 1: Forward Bend Test

Start by standing with your feet shoulder-width apart. Bend forward to touch your toes. Stand back up. This test could be indicative of a lower back spinal instability problem if any of the following occurred:

1. You felt a catch or a click in your back
2. You felt a twinge of sharp pain in your back
3. Your movement was not smooth, and it shifted from side to side
4. You needed to use your hands on your thighs to help you return to the standing position

Test 2: Painful Catch Test

Start by lying on your back. Lift both legs in the air and ensure that your knees are straight. Slowly return to the starting position. This test could be indicative of lower back spinal instability if any of the following occurred:

1. You felt a catch or a click in your back
2. You felt a twinge of sharp pain in your back
3. Your legs fall instantly or quickly because of the low back pain

Test 3: Stability Endurance Test in 90/90 Position

Start by lying on your back with support under your head, your knees bent, and your feet flat. Blow all your air out and flatten your lower back. Keeping this position, lift your legs in the air with your knees bent so that your hips and knees are at 90-degree angles. Continue breathing and keep the low back flat while you count. Stop counting and stop the test when any of the following occurs:

1. You are no longer able to maintain a flat back
2. Your legs start shaking
3. Your legs start to drop out of position because it's challenging to maintain
4. You begin to experience low back or hip pain

If you could not hold this position for 30 seconds before any of the above happened, this test may indicate a spinal stability issue.

Neck Self-Assessment Tests

Test 1: Backward Bend Test

Start by standing with your feet shoulder-width apart. Bend your head back slowly, then return your head to the starting position. This test could be indicative of a neck spinal instability problem if any of the following occurred:

1. You felt a catch or a click in your neck
2. You felt a twinge of sharp pain in your neck
3. Your head movement was not smooth or shifted from side to side
4. You needed to use your hand to bring your head back to the starting position

Test 2: Neck Flexion Endurance Test

Start by lying on your back with support under your head, your knees bent, and your feet flat. Blow all your air out and flatten your lower back. Tuck your chin in. Keeping this position, lift your head in the air 1-2 inches off the surface. Continue steady breathing and maintain chin tuck and head lift position while counting. Stop counting and stop the test when any of the following occurs:

1. You are no longer able to maintain the chin tuck
2. Your head and neck start shaking
3. Your head starts to drop out of position because it's challenging to maintain
4. You begin to experience neck pain

If you could not hold this position for 30 seconds before any of the above happened, this test may indicate a spinal stability issue.

Test 3: Neck Extension Endurance Test

Lying on your stomach with support under your forehead (folded towel). Tuck your chin in. Keeping this position, lift your head in the air 1-2 inches off the surface. Continue steady breathing and maintain chin tuck and head lift position while counting. Stop counting and stop the test when any of the following occurs:

1. You are no longer able to keep the chin tuck position
2. Your neck starts shaking
3. Your head starts to drop out of position because it's challenging to maintain
4. You begin to experience neck or back pain

If you could not hold this position for 30 seconds before any of the above happened, this test may indicate a spinal stability issue.

Stability Corrective Exercises

Deep spinal stability is fundamental to our postural stability and ability to move. So, training this fundamental spinal stability will improve your ability to withstand and manage the forces of everyday life. Everyone can benefit from these exercises, whether they have neck or back symptoms.

Although these exercises would benefit many of us, how an exercise is performed is important, especially when it comes to awareness-based or activation-based exercises like these. The best place to do them is with a trained professional in a clinical setting. If you attempt to do these exercises at home, pay attention to the quality, move slowly, and discontinue if they cause pain. With these exercises, you should feel muscle activity but not pain. If you have questions or reservations, seek a physical therapist, chiropractor, or personal trainer first to know the proper and safe way to perform them before you try on your own.

Keep these principles in mind when doing all these corrective activation exercises:[28]

1. Perform slowly. This will improve your deeper awareness and quality of the movement.

2. Maintain postural alignment. A parallel rib-pelvis relationship and spinal elongation are key to effectively engaging the stability system.

3. Maintain steady breathing. Don't hold your breath or breathe excessively.

4. Focus on the quality. Quality is better than quantity when it comes to this type of exercise.

5. Perform daily. The more you practice, the more proficient you become and the deeper awareness you create.

The first two exercises, Ribs Down Position with Diaphragmatic Breathing and Intra-abdominal Pressure with Exhalation, are fundamental. They should be mastered before performing the specific back and neck exercises. It usually takes 2-4 weeks for my patients to become proficient with the first two exercises.

Correct Positioning

3-Month-Old Supine Position

The position of these first two exercises is called the 3-month-old Supine Position because it correlates to the baby's position on its back at 3 months of age. The head should be supported by a small pillow or folded towel so that your neck is not extended back. The shoulders should be freely resting on the ground. The legs should be supported, keeping your hips and knees at 90 degrees (90/90 position). You can use a chair, couch, or bed to support your legs in this position. Your hips should be slightly open, so the knees are further apart than your feet.

Common Mistakes

Watch out for these common mistakes during any exercise performed in the 3-Month-Old Supine Position:

- Head and neck hyperextension
- Shoulders not in contact with the ground
- Lower rib position elevated
- Overactivity of the upper abdominals
- Stomach drawing in
- Stomach protruding out
- Lower back is not in contact with the ground

Exercise 1: Ribs Down with Diaphragmatic Breathing

The position of the lower rib cage in relation to the pelvis is critical for the optimal function of the diaphragm in breathing and stabilization. The relationship between the lower rib cage and the pelvis should be parallel (stacked on top of one another). This exercise improves this postural alignment and awareness.

Benefits of Ribs Down with Diaphragmatic Breathing

- Corrects the lower rib cage-to-pelvis alignment
- Improves awareness of this optimal alignment, which is key to being able to correct it in everyday life activities
- Improves rib cage and thoracic spine mobility
- Improves tone and function of muscles between the ribs
- Can alleviate back and neck pain while doing the exercise

How To Do Ribs Down with Diaphragmatic Breathing

1. Start in 3-Month-Old Supine Position: lying on your back with legs supported so your hips and knees are at 90 degrees (Table-Top or 90/90 position).

2. Lower your lower rib cage toward your pelvis to achieve the optimal parallel position to one another. Place your hands on your lower rib cage to feel the movement of the rib cage descending towards the ground or your pelvis.

The lower rib cage position can be achieved by performing any of the following.

- Exhale completely
- Exhale forcibly by making the "shhh" sound
- Sternal crunch by attempting to flatten your sternum towards the ground

3. Maintain this position as you perform diaphragmatic breathing. Breathe 360 degrees around your abdomen. Feel the breath go towards the lower abdomen, the side of the ribs, and the back—review the breathing chapter exercises for more detail.

4. Maintain the position as you inhale and reinforce the position as you exhale for 3-5 breath cycles. Then relax everything and repeat for the next set of 3-5 breaths. Perform 5 sets of 3-5 breaths.

Any prolonged or forced exhalation will bring the rib cage into a lower position, which is what you are trying to learn to recreate. Breathing into the position will maximize the diaphragmatic excursion, the soft tissue mobility around the rib cage and abdomen, and the rib cage mobility.

Exercise 2: Intra-abdominal Pressure with Exhalation

Benefits of Intra-abdominal Pressure with Exhalation

- Creates the deeper spinal stability that supports and elongates the spine

- Improves the awareness of muscle activity necessary to create intra-abdominal pressure
- Improves the coordination and control of creating the pressure while breathing (without holding the breath)
- Supports the lower back and spine
- Addresses the postural stability necessary to address the long-term solution of postural and muscle imbalances
- Can alleviate back and neck pain while doing the exercise

How to do Intra-abdominal Pressure with Exhalation

1. Start in 3-Month-Old Supine Position: lying on your back with legs supported, so your hips and knees are at 90 degrees (same position as the previous exercise). You can use a chair, couch, or bed to support your legs in this position. Your hips should be slightly open, so the knees are further apart than your feet.

2. Lower your lower rib cage toward your pelvis to achieve their optimal parallel position to one another. Place your hands on your lower rib cage to feel the movement of the rib cage descending towards the ground or your pelvis (same as the previous exercise).

3. Maintain this position as you perform diaphragmatic breathing. Place your fingertips in any of these locations:
    - Between belly button and pubic bone
    - Outside of lower ribs

- Lower back between the 12th rib and pelvis

4. Inhale by breathing into your fingertips, and then maintain this outward pressure feeling as you exhale. Your abdomen will naturally recoil, fall, or give as you exhale but attempt to keep it inflated outward. Don't let your belly drop. Think about inflating a balloon as you breathe in, and keep that balloon inflated as you breathe out. What you are creating is intra-abdominal pressure.

5. Maintain this pressure for 3-5 breath cycles, depending on what you can maintain. Then relax and repeat for the next set of 3-5 breaths. Work up to 5 sets of 5 breaths.

Special Modifications with Intra-abdominal Pressure with Exhalation

Blow Up a Balloon

The Intra-abdominal Pressure with Exhalation Exercise may be difficult for some who can get their lower rib cage in the correct position but can't maintain the outward pressure as they exhale. If that is the case, modify the exercise by blowing into a balloon. The same setup as the exercise described above, but you hold a balloon to your mouth with one hand and use your other hand to feel the correct activation.

To perform, inhale through the nose and then attempt to blow up the balloon as you exhale. Repeat for 3-5 exhalations. Even if you can't blow up the balloon, you will feel the proper intra-abdominal pressure activation as you attempt to exhale into the balloon. Ditch the balloon once you can do without it.

Release Extra Tension

It is common for people to feel increased tension in their neck, shoulders, and chest as they do this exercise. Often it is because they are trying too hard and overcompensating. You only need to meet the demands of the movement. Maintain pressure and breathe without creating tension in the neck and shoulders.

Keep Your Buttocks Out of It

Another common mistake is to squeeze the buttocks or tilt the pelvis to flatten the lower back to the ground. This is usually due to difficulty bringing the rib cage down to meet the pelvis. If this is the case, place a small pillow or folded towel under your pelvis and hips. This will raise the pelvis higher and thus will make it easier for your rib cage to align itself with the pelvis in a parallel relationship.

Progressions with Emphasis for the Back

The following two exercises are a progression of the stabilization activation exercises that are specific to improving stability for the back, but they are also helpful in enhancing stability in the neck. Both exercises are performed in the 3-Month-Old Supine position.

Exercise 3: Intra-abdominal Pressure with Isometric Hip Flexion

This exercise is an excellent progression for reinforcing intra-abdominal pressure activation and is especially useful if you are having difficulty creating intra-abdominal pressure. Plus, it shares all the benefits of Intra-abdominal Pressure with Exhalation exercise.

How to perform Intra-abdominal Pressure with Isometric Hip Flexion

1. Start in 3-Month-Old Supine Position: lying on your back with legs supported so that your hips and knees are at 90 degrees.

2. Lower your lower rib cage toward your pelvis to achieve their optimal parallel position to one another. Place your hands on your lower rib cage so you can feel the movement of the rib cage descending toward the ground or your pelvis. Maintain this position as you perform diaphragmatic breathing.

3. Place the palms of both hands on your front lower thigh just above your knee. Breathe into your abdomen 360 degrees around. As you exhale, push your hands into your thighs (with approximately 25% effort) as you maintain intra-abdominal pressure.

4. Maintain this pressure for 3-5 breath cycles. Then relax and repeat for the next set of 3-5. Work up to 5 sets of 5 breaths.

Exercise 4: Intra-abdominal Pressure with Leg Unloading

This progression of the stabilization exercises in the 3-Month-Old Supine Position begins to teach the coordination of moving a limb while maintaining intra-abdominal pressure. In addition to all the previous benefits, this exercise is good for hip flexor overactivity and strains, sacroiliac joint dysfunction, and instability with hip flexion movements (e.g., walking, stair climbing, running, hiking, etc.).

How to do Intra-abdominal Pressure with Leg Unloading

1. Start in 3-Month-Old Supine Position: lying on your back with legs supported so that your hips and knees are at 90 degrees.

2. Lower your lower rib cage toward your pelvis to achieve their optimal parallel position to one another. Place your hands on your lower rib cage so you can feel the movement of the rib cage descending toward the ground or toward your pelvis. Maintain this position as you perform diaphragmatic breathing.

3. Place your fingertips in any of these locations:

    - Between belly button and pubic bone
    - Outside of lower ribs
    - Lower back between the 12th rib and pelvis

4. Inhale by breathing into your fingertips. Once ready, maintain this feeling of outward pressure and exhale while you slowly lift one leg off the support toward your head. Finish your exhalation. Inhale, and then exhale while maintaining pressure and slowly lowering your leg to the starting position. Repeat for the other leg.

5. Once finished with one set of unloading each leg, relax entirely and repeat for 3-5 sets. Work up to 5 sets of alternate legs.

Modification:

Once proficient with unloading each leg independently, you can progress to unloading both legs. Repeat the exercise as prescribed with the addition of raising the second leg in the air after the first leg is already unloaded in the air. The final position is both legs unloaded with the legs in the air as you maintain pressure and breathing.

Progressions with Emphasis for the Neck

The following two exercises are a progression of the stabilization activation exercises specific to improving neck stability. Both exercises are performed in the 3-Month-Old Supine position.

Exercise 5: Intra-abdominal Pressure with Chin Tuck

This exercise is an excellent introduction to deep neck stability activation in conjunction with intra-abdominal pressure activation. I give this exercise to all my patients dealing with neck and postural issues. It is also a prerequisite for the second exercise, Intra-abdominal Pressure with Head Lift.

How to perform Intra-abdominal Pressure with Chin Tuck

1. Start in 3-Month-Old Supine Position: lying on your back with legs supported, so your hips and knees are at 90 degrees.

2. Lower your lower rib cage toward your pelvis to achieve their optimal parallel position to one another. Place your hands on your lower rib cage to feel the movement of the rib cage descending toward the ground or toward your pelvis. Maintain this position as you perform diaphragmatic breathing.

3. Breathe into your abdomen 360 degrees around. As you exhale, slightly tuck your chin in as if you were nodding yes while maintaining intra-abdominal pressure.

4. Maintain this pressure for 3-5 breath cycles. Then relax and repeat for the next set of 3-5 sets. Work up to 5 sets of 5 breaths.

Modifications and Special Considerations:

- Do not overdo the chin tuck movement. If you try too hard, you will overcompensate with your superficial neck muscles, which is not ideal. Meet the demand of the exercise, no more and no less.

- If you have difficulty creating a chin tuck movement, your neck may be hyperextended. Ensure that you have adequate or additional head support (folded towel) and repeat. You should find it easier to create the chin movement.

- Be sure you are not creating additional neck and shoulder tension as you perform the exercise by lifting your chest upward or shrugging your shoulders toward your head. The chest and sternum should be down flat, and the shoulders should be fixed downward away from your ears.

Exercise 6: Intra-Abdominal Pressure with Head Lift

This exercise is a progression of deep neck stability activation in conjunction with intra-abdominal pressure activation in a 3-month-old supine position. It may take several weeks of proficiency with the previous exercise (Intra-abdominal Pressure with Chin Tuck) before you can perform this exercise optimally.

How to Perform Intra-Abdominal Pressure with Head Lift

1. Start in 3-Month-Old Supine Position: lying on your back with legs supported so that your hips and knees are at 90 degrees.

2. Lower your lower rib cage toward your pelvis to achieve their optimal parallel position to one another. Place your hands on your lower rib cage so you can feel the movement of the rib cage descending toward the ground or your pelvis. Maintain this position as you perform diaphragmatic breathing.

3. Breathe into your abdomen 360 degrees around. As you exhale, slightly tuck your chin in as if you were nodding 'Yes,' then lift your head 1-2 inches while maintaining intra-abdominal pressure.

4. Maintain this pressure and position for 3-5 breath cycles. Then relax and repeat for the next set of 3-5 breaths. Work up to 5 sets of 5 breaths.

Modifications and Special Considerations:

- Do not attempt to poke your head upward or flex your neck by bringing your chin to your chest. The head and neck should lift as a unit together with the sternum as the stable base. Maintain the spinal elongation as if someone were pulling the top of your head with a string.

- Be aware of the stable progression of the exercise. Feel and imagine that the head is lifting from the elongation of the neck with the chin tuck because of the stability created below. The movement of the head is the natural consequence of the stability you have created. Your neck should feel like it is floating upward with little effort.

- If you have difficulty with excessive shaking or inability to perform without pain or discomfort, go back to the previous exercise.

- Be sure you are not creating additional neck and shoulder tension as you perform the exercise by lifting your chest upward or shrugging your shoulders toward your head. The chest and sternum should be down flat, and the shoulders should be fixed downward away from your ears.

Conclusion

These six exercises are fundamental to improving your innate ability to create stability and optimize your movement. Perform these exercises daily, slowly, and with good quality. If you do, there is no doubt you will improve the coordination and the endurance of your deep stability system. The result will be less accessory muscle tension, less painful recurrent episodes, and improved posture. This could be the best thing you ever do for your spinal health.

CHAPTER 8

Postural Stability in Everyday Life

"Nothing is permanent about our behavior patterns except our belief that they are so."

Moshé Feldenkrais

Awareness of Alignment, Breath, and Intra-abdominal Pressure

This is my overarching goal for the people I help—*improved quality of movement and dynamic stability so that they can physically function and perform at their best in their everyday lives and protect themselves from reinjury with the ultimate goal of self-reliance in the self-management of their physical neuromusculoskeletal problems.*

One of the most challenging and possibly more critical aspects of achieving this goal is incorporating the clinical lessons and exercises into everyday life. Patients often ask:

- How do I do this while I'm sitting at my desk?

- How do I do this during my exercise routine?

- I can create pressure when I'm on my back doing the exercises, but why can't I seem to do it while I am standing?

- Do I have to stay constantly engaged, 24-7?

Whenever I get asked these questions, I explain a concept regarding how we learn new motor control skills. In learning to control or coordinate movement, people typically go through four stages of learning:

1. **Unconsciously Incompetent:** you are not aware of the coordinated movement, nor are you able to perform the movement

2. **Consciously Incompetent:** you have an awareness and understanding of the coordinated movement, but you are unable to perform the coordinated movement on your own

3. **Consciously Competent:** you have awareness and understanding of the coordination movement, and you can perform the coordinated movement on your own with deliberate effort.

4. **Unconsciously Competent:** you have an unconscious awareness and understanding of the coordinated movement so that you can perform the coordinated movement intuitively without thinking about it or trying to do so.

The goal is to become unconsciously competent in maintaining good postural alignment and stability while walking, driving, exercising, gardening, etc., without conscious effort. To get there, you need improved body awareness, training and feedback, and initial mindfulness during activities of everyday living. It takes time, but the results are worth it.

Body Awareness

Body awareness is the key! Having some basic knowledge of ideal postural stability and its relation to your neck or back problem is essential. You need to feel in your body where you are in space and how to coordinate your breathing, your stability, and your movements. Fortunately, your initial body awareness improves as you learn how to correct your posture, restore your optimal breath, and optimize your postural spinal stability.

Improving your body awareness trumps the knowledge of how your body works. For some, understanding and awareness come quickly. For others, it is much more challenging. In my practice, I employ various ways of improving people's ability to perceive and modify coordinated body movements. Some methods don't require verbal instructions or understanding by the patient but rather work through manual feedback and stimulation.

Training and Feedback

Once initial body awareness has been improved, training and feedback are necessary to advance further. Enhancing and cementing awareness of optimal posture, breathing, and stabilization is only possible through the repetition of postural correction and the consistency of a postural stabilization exercise program. This requires feedback over time so that optimally coordinated patterns are adequately instilled.

Although some pick up on the exercises quickly, no one ever gets it after one training session. It requires periodic review with someone who knows what to look for, and it also involves the progression of the exercises over time based on the person's needs and goals.

Mindfulness in Daily Life Activities

Once the optimal stabilization has been sufficiently trained and there is a specific competence level, awareness and correction in daily activities are possible. During any movement or physical activity in life, the following conditions need to be met—correct postural alignment, steady abdominal breathing, and intra-abdominal pressure that meets the demands of the movement or physical activity. It's both simple and challenging.

It requires some attention and presence at the moment. If you are rushing around, you won't be mindful enough to be aware of your posture and how you are doing things. Easier said than done, but it is possible to become unconsciously competent with a consistent focus on mindfulness and repeated self-correction.

The Needs of Daily Activities

As I move through the rest of the chapter, I will discuss what's necessary for different activities of daily living in more detail. I may risk sounding like a broken record here because the same basic principles apply to any movement or physical activity. In everything you do, the following need to be addressed:

Step 1: Postural Alignment

We covered postural alignment in Chapter 5. Stacked posture, with pelvis over feet, chest over the pelvis, and head over the chest. Maintenance of the spine's normal curvature, especially of the lumbar spine. Spinal length and elongation. Parallel, stacked position of the lower rib cage to the pelvis. That's step number one!

Step 2: Steady Diaphragmatic Breathing

Steady breathing should be maintained throughout the movement or activity. No holding of the breath. No excessive breathing. The breath should be low in the stomach and not in the chest.

Step 3: Maintenance of Intra-abdominal Pressure

All physical activities and movements require some intra-abdominal pressure, though activities vary in how much pressure is needed. Opening a light door requires less than opening a heavy door. Lifting 50lbs off the ground requires more than bending at the bathroom sink to brush your teeth. Maintenance of intra-abdominal pressure that meets the movement's or activity's demands will protect the spine, prevent possible injury, and maximize the function of our limbs.

Sitting

It's a sign of the times that sitting is essential to talk about when it comes to our physical health. Everyone is now aware of the danger of sitting. It's talked about on mainstream television, tons of books have covered it, and everyone has an opinion on it, especially those who decide to give it up entirely and go to a standing desk, which is especially beneficial for the standing desk industry and maybe for podiatrists and orthotics companies, too.

Ironically, sitting doesn't require a whole lot of dynamic postural stability. Moving requires much more postural stability than static sitting, but we still need to fight gravity, and sitting is more compressive on the spine than standing is.

I don't want to discuss the ill effects of sitting. The laundry list of potential dangers is long, as all those other books attest. But the reality is that sitting is a big part of our lives, whether we like it or not. We sit in our cars, at our computers, and for much of our passive entertainment. Two years after the start of the COVID pandemic, we are sitting even more than we ever did for our meetings and get-togethers. It doesn't have to be a problem; you don't have to eliminate it completely. But it is imperative to get it right.

Postural Alignment in Sitting

Postural alignment is the key to sitting because optimal breathing and postural stability are impossible without it. Without the stacked alignment of the rib cage over the pelvis, the diaphragm cannot fully function in its respiratory and stabilization function. This is especially crucial because we tend to sit for long periods.

For a detailed explanation of setting yourself up for optimal postural alignment in sitting, look back at the sitting posture correction exercise in Chapter 5. Still, I will summarize some key points that will set you up for an optimal alignment.

First, your hips should ideally be at the level of or higher than your knees. This will ensure a neutral pelvis position and maintain the normal curve inward of the lumbar spine, which sets up an ideal alignment for the rest of the spine. If you are sitting at a desk chair, regular chair, or stool and your hips are below the level of your knees, raise the chair so that the hip level is higher than your knees. If the chair you are sitting in does not raise and lower, raise the height by sitting on a cushion or pillow.

Second, your feet should be in contact with the ground. If raising your chair height results in your feet no longer touching the floor, then you will need a footstool. Having your feet fully stable and supported on the ground is important for adding stability that unloads some forces on our spine.

Third, find and maintain your neutral pelvis position. Overcorrect (arch) your pelvis forward and then return to find the neutral pelvis position (where you feel most comfortable and like you are sitting on your sit bones). Use lumbar support to maintain this position. There are plenty on the market, but anything will do in a pinch (jacket, towel, cushion, etc.). You must consciously maintain this neutral pelvis position when you can't sit back in the chair with support. If you aren't careful, you will invariably slip back into a backward pelvis position and lose your optimal spinal alignment, resulting in excessive stress and strain on your neck and back muscles, joints, ligaments, discs, and fascia. Maintaining the ideal pelvis alignment is critical for prolonged sitting situations.

Breathing in Sitting

Now that you have your ideal postural alignment in sitting, it's time to focus on your breath. Steady, slow, full belly breaths are the way to go. It will be more challenging for some to fully belly breathe while sitting than lying on their back in the 90/90 or tabletop position. This is because there are forces at play in sitting that we don't have to deal with lying on our back with our legs supported, mainly the forces of gravity and muscle imbalances. Remember to keep your chest quiet (minimal to no elevation) and feel the breath going down toward your pelvis and 360 degrees around your waist. Breathing into your waistband is a perfect visualization.

Intra-Abdominal Pressure in Sitting

After focusing on steady, slow belly breathing, you can shift your focus to maintaining intra-abdominal pressure. Place your hands on your belly to get feedback and feel what's happening. You can place your thumbs in the backside of your trunk (there is a slight depression below your ribs and above your pelvis where you can stick your thumbs) and your fingers on the side of your belly or lower belly area. Continue breathing into these areas. To create intra-abdominal pressure, you should aim to maintain pressure against your thumb and fingers as you exhale. Focus on relaxing your neck and shoulders. Keep your breath low. Don't hold your breath, and don't excessively breathe. You should feel that your posture is automatically growing taller. This is postural stability in sitting!

As you become more competent in this position, try to add external factors such as talking or movement. Start talking while trying to maintain the pressure. This is not as easy as it seems. Try keeping the pressure while turning your neck side to side. Try holding the pressure while slowly lifting one arm and then the other. Continue slowly and steadily breathing throughout without tensing up different body parts. Try maintaining the pressure while reaching out in front of you, hinging at your hips, and keeping your postural alignment. Now your postural stability is dynamic.

Helpful Tips for Sitting

- Set up an ergonomic workstation and buy an ergonomic desk chair if you spend a long time doing desk work or computer work.
- Raise the height of your chair or raise your hips using a cushion to ensure your hips are higher than your knees.
- If your feet are no longer touching the ground, use a footstool.
- Use lumbar support to help maintain ideal postural alignment.
- Set a timer every 20-30 minutes to take a break.
- During the break, stand up, walk around, do some simple stretches, or drink a glass of water.

- Upon return to sitting, run through the 3 phases of optimal posture and stability in sitting:
    1. Set up optimal postural alignment
    2. Awareness of breath (5-10 breathes)
    3. Create intra-abdominal pressure (3-5 breaths)

The goal is not to create abdominal pressure maximally and constantly while you are sitting. The goal is to train the sense of your body position and alignment, the awareness of your breath, and the maintenance of the intra-abdominal pressure in this sitting position with and without movement. The more you do this, the more you will feel and know the postural stability demands of sitting, and the more you will improve your postural stamina and endurance.

Standing

If the time spent sitting has increased over the years, you might think we are not spending as much time standing. While that may be true for some, it's certainly not true for everyone. Many people must stand long hours for their job, and some have adopted a standing workstation. Even if you sit for work, there are times that you may find yourself standing for a period, as when standing in a line, at your kid's game, or in the kitchen preparing a meal.

Prolonged standing can pose specific challenges to our musculoskeletal system. Some spinal conditions such as spinal stenosis, spondylolisthesis, and systemic hypermobility may limit standing to 5-10 minutes before the onset of symptoms. For people with significant postural and muscle imbalances, standing for 30 minutes to cook dinner or a couple of hours for a shift at work can be uncomfortable and painful.

The pain or discomfort from prolonged standing can present as foot pain, knee pain, hip pain, low back pain, or neck pain. Which body part decides to complain is dependent on many factors, but it will invariably be an area where the body's muscles, ligaments, joints, or nerves are dealing with a load and a strain that they cannot tolerate.

Thus, it might present as a plantar fasciitis type pain, knee joint pain, or sacroiliac joint pain. Or the nerves might be the primary pain driver, especially when prolonged standing causes the legs to ache or the arms to feel heavy. The spinal nerves become compressed and prevent an adequate blood supply. This sensitizes the nerves, resulting in referred pain that travels down an extremity and further sensitizes muscle trigger points.

The solution is to improve postural spinal stability while standing. We do that through awareness of postural alignment, restoration of optimal breathing, and maintenance of intra-abdominal pressure.

Postural Alignment in Standing

A few essential factors make standing different from sitting for optimal postural alignment. For one, the support base is your feet rather than your pelvis. Second, there is the less available range in your spine because the length of the hip flexors and hamstrings limits the mobility of the pelvis. The adjustment you made to the pelvis in sitting will be more limited and more minor of a factor in standing.

Start with your base of support to get to an optimal postural alignment while standing. The first thing to do is be aware of your feet width. If you stand with your feet less than hip-width apart, your base of support will be too narrow, resulting in more body effort to maintain balance. A broader support base, somewhere between hip-width and shoulder-width apart, is better. Find a distance that feels stable to you.

Next, focus on bearing weight through the base of your big toe, the base of the little toe, and the heel. Be sure to maintain your arch without losing those contact points. Then elongate your spine. It should feel as though you are growing taller through the crown of your head while keeping your lower ribs in place. Be conscious of your overall postural alignment, keeping your pelvis stacked over your feet, your chest stacked over your pelvis, and your head stacked over your chest. For a more detailed overview of optimal standing postural correction, refer to Chapter 5.

Breathing in Standing

Once you have corrected your standing postural alignment, you can shift your focus to your breathing. The goal is to maintain your postural alignment while your awareness is on steady abdominal breathing. You can place your hands in the three focus areas to encourage a breath that is 360 degrees around. These are the lower abdominal area, the side of the ribs, and the back outside aspect of the lower ribs and back. Focus on breathing into each location for several breaths.

The excursion of your breath will also be more limited in the standing than the sitting position, so you may find it more difficult to notice your abdominal breathing. Remember not to attempt a big breath, as that will likely encourage a breath higher in the chest. This is a common side effect of people trying too hard to breathe correctly. The result is the opposite of what you are aiming for. Practicing in front of a mirror can be helpful, as it gives visual feedback on where you are breathing.

Intra-abdominal Pressure in Standing

Now that you have some awareness of your breath while standing create intra-abdominal pressure by maintaining the pressure out 360 degrees as you inhale and exhale. Take it nice and easy. Feel the outward pressure in all directions, like air pushing out from the inside of a balloon. If done right, you should feel that your posture is growing taller. Practice for several breaths.

Helpful Tips in Standing

- Be mindful of your support base and ensure it is not too narrow. Aim for hip-width to shoulder-width apart, whichever feels most stable to you. A staggered position with one foot in front of the other in a broader stance will also help dissipate the forces through your legs and spine.

- Wear orthotics or good supportive shoes while standing for prolonged periods, especially if you have flat feet or your feet are over-pronated. This will ensure that you set yourself up to maintain a better alignment kinematic chain through the lower body. I recommend Vasyli orthotics and Vionic shoes and sandals for my patients, but there are other good orthotic and shoe solutions out there as well.

- If you are forced to stand for a long time, shift your weight gently from side to side. This will make standing a bit more dynamic and engage your lower body to be more active, lessening the stress on your spine.

- If you are going to utilize a standing desk, do not go from sitting for hours to standing for hours at a time. Your body is not likely to be prepared for that, which may cause other problems. Instead, gradually shift over time so that it is not so dramatic a change. For instance, add standing for 1 hour a day for a week, then change to 2 hours a day for a week, and so on.

- If you opt for a standing desk, I recommend a setup that allows the transition to and from a sitting desk configuration to a standing desk one. You will be better off spending some of the day sitting and standing rather than your entire workday doing one or the other.

- As with sitting, be mindful not to spend too much time standing still for too long of a time at work. Take breaks every 30 minutes, walk around, stretch, or grab some water before returning to your standing desk to resume your work.

The goal is not to be able to stand for an unlimited amount of time. Instead, it is to correct your standing posture, be aware of your breath, and improve the endurance of your postural stability in standing. Then you will be able to access this stability when the demand increases.

For instance, you may find that your neck or back starts to fatigue and ache while standing for activities such as washing the dishes, preparing a meal, or waiting in a grocery line. We all do these activities in our daily lives; being unable to do so easily affects your quality of life. But if you can improve your ability to stand in the moment, you will increase your standing capacity and stamina, meaning there will be less pain and fatigue when life requires you to stand.

Walking

We walk every day. We walk to our car, walk into the store, walk around at work, walk our dogs, walk for exercise, and walk for recreational activities like traveling and sightseeing. Compared to sitting and standing, walking is dynamic—in constant motion. So, it's not as demanding on the body from a static postural standpoint, but it can present its own set of problems, especially walking for a prolonged period.

If you have a postural stability problem affected by walking, it could present in many ways during or after a long walk. Increased neck or back pain. Deep ache or a feeling of pressure or heaviness in one arm or both arms. The same can be true for the legs. Maintaining an upright posture may feel challenging. However, you might feel it; poor postural and spinal stability can result in irritated spinal nerves and overloaded muscles that start to talk to you. The earlier you begin to feel these symptoms during a walk, the worse the condition is likely to be.

However, once you have built up sufficient stability through the exercises and greater awareness of your posture and breathing, walking is an excellent initial physical activity that you can use to practice dynamic postural stability. At first, it may be more challenging to coordinate postural correction, awareness of breath, and maintenance of intra-abdominal pressure while you are moving. But practicing the exercises and remembering the principles in this book will help you improve your postural stability with walking.

Postural Alignment with Walking

First, ensure that you have good, supportive walking shoes and use orthotics if needed. If you have flat feet and walk in sandals or shoes with little arch support, you ask for trouble. If you are under 18, you may get away with it, but if you have lived enough years to have physical problems, you won't for long.

Next, focus on correcting your postural alignment while you are walking. It does not need to be as systematic as in standing posture.

Keep it simple. Feel the sensation of growing taller through the crown of your head while keeping your ribs down, chest open, shoulders down, and chin slightly tucked in. If you fix your posture by squeezing your shoulder blades back and sticking your chest out, you will undoubtedly be arching your lower back and compromising the lower rib and pelvis relationship. So, the key is to grow taller without lifting your lower ribs toward your chest and head. You can do all of this while you are walking. It is a subtle feeling and something to focus on internally; no one will perceive you are doing it.

Breathing with Walking

Now that your postural alignment is ideal, you can start thinking about breathing correctly. Breathe in through the nose and feel the expansion of the breath low in the belly and not in the chest. Remember to feel the breath going down toward the lower abdominals and pelvis, out into the sides and back. Don't try too hard, as that will only encourage a big breath in your chest and neck. If you are not in great shape, you might find that you are using some accessory breathing muscles in your neck to meet the demands of your walk. Working on diaphragmatic breathing will help you meet the oxygen demands more efficiently. Guided walking meditation is another great tool to use. Regardless of how you do it, walking is an excellent time to focus on your breath.

Intra-abdominal Pressure with Walking

You have brought awareness to your posture and breath, and now it's time to add the final piece—create a little pressure. As you focus on your diaphragmatic breathing, create the intra-abdominal pressure by gently pushing outward as you are breathing. If done right, it will feel like your posture is straightening up further and creating stability from the inside out. As in other physical activities, you only need enough pressure to meet the movement's demands. In the case of walking, that is enough stability to fight gravity and propel your limbs to move you forward. Too much will cause you to feel stiff and robotic. Too little will leave you feeling loosey-goosey. Find the level of stability that makes you feel that you are solid and tall but fluid and free with the movement of your arms and legs. It is a beautiful feeling of freedom and comfort when you get it just right.

Helpful Tips for Walking

- Wear good supportive shoes and orthotics if you have poor foot support.

- Don't walk with too narrow of a base of support. Walk with your feet hip-width apart.

- Grow tall. Think about a string pulling the crown of your head toward the sky.

- Maintain your postural alignment while you grow tall. No arching of the back, no chest up, no shoulders up, no head bent back. Keep your ribs down, chest open, shoulders down, and chin slightly tucked.

- Breathe in through your nose as best you can and feel the low abdominal breathing pattern, not a chest and neck breathing pattern.

- Find enough stability to fight gravity and propel you forward while allowing for the fluid movement of your arms and legs.

- Use your arms. They help to give you momentum. Walking is a contra-lateral pattern, meaning your opposite arm and leg move simultaneously forward. Practice this if you lack this coordination.

As with sitting and standing, you don't have to obsess about all this while walking. Just bring your awareness to it from time to time. The more attention you have around it and the more you play with it, the more you will improve your postural stability with walking over time. The result will be more efficient walking, longer walking distances before symptoms arise, and more stability for those unexpected moments when a dog pulls on the leash or you lose your balance on uneven terrain.

Functional Activities

Functional activities are all the functional movements we do daily without much thought. Examples are turning in bed, transferring from a lying to a sitting position, standing from a sitting position, bending, squatting, lifting, getting in and out of a car, etc.

These functional activities typically involve multiple body parts and include transitioning from one position to another or from one activity to another. They are purposeful body movements. We usually don't give these activities much thought because they have ingrained in our bodies and nervous system. Until, of course, we can't do them. Then, we quickly realize just how important they are.

Our functional activities are typically hindered when we experience pain, lose mobility, lose stability and strength, or lose coordination.

If you have ever suffered from an acute painful back or neck episode, you know how pain can affect your functional activities. Simple activities such as turning in bed, getting up from a chair, or bending down to pick something up can be painful and limited. The spasm and pain from an acute neck or back episode can be so limiting that it affects all movements and the ability to withstand positions like sitting and standing. Thankfully, this acute phase typically only lasts a few days to a week.

A loss of functional mobility could include being unable to squat down low or get up from the floor. A loss of mobility and flexibility in your spine, hips, and knees can be the main limiting factor. The old saying goes, "If you don't use it, you lose it." If you are not accustomed to squatting low to the ground or are not consistently crouching down to the ground, you may lose the functional mobility to do it.

Losing stability and strength can also affect your functional ability, causing difficulties transitioning from one position to another, such as when getting up from a chair, returning from a bent forward position, or difficulty carrying and lifting items. The cause is often inadequate postural and spinal stability due to a history of long-standing pain, functional limitations, and avoidance of physical activity. Working on the underlying core stability can do wonders in restoring a person's ability to perform functional activities.

Lack of coordination can also substantially affect our ability to move functionally. If you have ever known anyone who has suffered a stroke or a traumatic brain injury, you have witnessed how difficult it can be for that person to get out of a car, sit down in a chair, or bend over to pick something up from the ground. Their nervous system has been damaged, affecting their motor patterns and motor control. Poor coordination can also be compromised in people without nervous system damage. Long-standing pain will affect our coordination. Avoiding the activities and aging also affect it. Sometimes, the most meaningful sessions with my patients are simply working on coordinating some of these seemingly simple, everyday functional activities.

Postural Alignment with Functional Activities

The details of postural alignment as previously reviewed in sitting, standing, and walking are all the same here. You still want to bring awareness and correct your postural alignment before initiating any physical activity. Then be aware of maintaining that postural alignment as you transition through the physical activity. This is different from just thinking about your postural alignment while sitting, standing, and walking, where the alignment stays relatively constant. You want to maintain your postural alignment throughout the physical activity with functional activities. For instance, maintain optimal spinal alignment and lower ribs-pelvis position while getting in and out of a chair, bending to reach for something, or squatting to pick something up. For the most part, if you can think about hinging through your hips rather than bending through your spine, you will give yourself the best chance of maintaining your postural alignment.

Breathing with Functional Activities

Awareness of breath is not as critical while dynamically moving through functional activities. However, taking a second and being aware of your breath is still a good idea before starting the physical activity. It will help keep you centered and focused before the movement. It will also prepare you to create the intra-abdominal pressure requirements of the activity. Perhaps the most important lesson is to avoid holding your breath during the activity. If all you do is catch yourself holding your breath, that is an insightful and helpful recognition.

Intra-abdominal Pressure with Functional Activities

Creating and maintaining intra-abdominal pressure while moving through physical activities is beneficial for anyone trying to improve their spinal and postural stability. It improves your awareness and trains your deeper proprioception of the stability requirements to perform certain activities. It is helpful to feel the differences in the stability requirements of rolling on your side from your back compared to reaching for a glass in the overhead cupboard or bending down to lift a 25lb box off the floor. The key is to maintain the optimal pressure throughout the physical activity movement based on the demands of that movement—no more and no less.

This awareness and training are easier said than done, but you can call upon your inner child when learning how to do it. The child does not know what stability demands are required to move from a sitting to a crawling position or from a half-kneeling to a standing position. They feel the stability requirements needed to maintain the starting position, then attempt to move, regulating that postural stability throughout the attempted movement. They fail at first because they don't necessarily have the capacity, but through the process of trying, failing, and trying again, they eventually figure it out.

Daily Life Activities

The key points to improving your postural and spinal stability in everyday life are awareness and attention to your postural alignment, breathing, and inner stability. There is no better way to practice this than in daily activities.

Daily activities cover everything from brushing your teeth, getting dressed, cooking, house cleaning, and driving. If you wish to transition from conscious incompetence to conscious competence, paying attention while doing the mundane tasks of everyday life will give you plenty of opportunities to do so. Over time, it will deepen your awareness and develop your stability as you take on more challenging physical demands and tasks.

However, daily activities can be problematic for those with postural and spinal stability problems. It's not uncommon for people to complain of neck and back pain when cooking, house cleaning, or driving. Not being able to maintain activity for an extended period can take a real toll on your life. It is hard to prepare a meal if you must stop to take breaks while the dish is cooking on the stove. If vacuuming and cleaning cause back pains, you may be forced to hire a cleaner to avoid it. And those vacations become a lot harder to take if you can't tolerate sitting in the car for more than a few minutes.

It is wiser to attempt to improve your ability to do these daily life activities over giving them up altogether. You don't want to lose your ability to function; you want to improve upon it. Taking the time to be mindful of how you do these daily activities and tasks can make all the difference.

Let's look at five examples of daily activities that you can use to bring awareness to the postural and spinal stability required.

Brushing Teeth

For most people, the time spent brushing their teeth is rarely problematic. But if you have an acute episode of back or neck pain, even this simple task can be excruciating. If you are someone who tends to bend over the sink to brush your teeth, pay close attention to your body and what it is telling you. You may notice that your neck or back is tensing up or feeling uncomfortable as you continue to brush. It is most likely due to a poor postural alignment, resulting in the muscles and ligaments becoming overworked and strained.

The solution is to stagger your feet, one in front of the other, find your optimal postural alignment, and bend through your hips like a hinge rather than curling through your spine. It should feel like you are sticking your butt out slightly. Now you can maintain an optimal spinal alignment while minimizing the stress on your neck and back. Also, examine your breathing pattern. Is it high or low? Is it deep or shallow? Measure how much stability it takes to maintain this posture. You can also place your hand on the counter for additional support.

Getting Dressed

Getting dressed is another mundane daily task we usually don't think about unless we can't physically do it. The next time you get dressed, take your time and be aware of how you are doing it.

How do you slip on your underwear, shorts, or pants? Do you sit to slip each leg through, or do you stand and balance on one leg to slip the other leg through? How stable do you feel when standing on one leg while getting dressed? If you don't balance your leg, when did you transition to sitting instead? How do you slip your shirt on? Do you always put one arm in first? Which one? Do you do it in an awkward way to avoid pain? How about bending down to put on your socks and shoes? Do you sit for this? Is this an easy task or a difficult one? These are all important questions to bring awareness to your postural stability while dressing.

If you are having trouble, the solution is to start with good postural alignment and bring awareness to your breathing and inner stability. Try to maintain this awareness as you shift your weight to balance on one leg. Keep your back straight as you bend down to put on your socks and shoes. The physical demands to dress are not that considerable, so the stability requirements will not be that considerable, especially since this task tends to be short-lived. But even so, bringing awareness to how you get dressed will reinforce your understanding of how to maintain postural integrity throughout your body. This can be very powerful and cement a much deeper knowledge within your body of what it means to be stable.

House Cleaning

I'm guessing this is not a favorite daily task for most people. I certainly don't enjoy doing the dishes, but since I have become more mindful, cleaning the dishes has turned into an introspective and purposeful task. A combination of static and dynamic forces is at play while doing the dishes, vacuuming, or making the bed. For example, while doing the dishes, you may need to maintain a position for some time while rinsing dishes at the sink, and you also need dynamic movements to unload and load the dishwasher. Vacuuming is dynamic, and it can be done in a sound way to reduce stress and strain.

Pay attention to your body alignment as you work over the sink, bend and turn your body to load the dishwasher, or raise glasses and dishware above your head to place them in the cupboard. Optimize your posture while hinging at your hips to vacuum. Move the vacuum by shifting your weight from the back leg to the front leg, not just through your arms and shoulders. Create intra-abdominal pressure while vacuuming and feel the additional stability it provides, minimizing excessive stress and tension through other parts of your body. Who would have thought that house cleaning could be so therapeutic?

Cooking

Like house cleaning, cooking is another daily activity that varies in its postural stability demands. Some activities are more static, such as standing to chop ingredients on the cutting board. Others are more dynamic, such as moving a heavy saucepan from the stove to the sink and back to boil water for cooking pasta.

You can bring attention to your posture, breathing, and stability while cooking. Create that intra-abdominal pressure just before and during lifting that heavy saucepan. Maintain an optimal standing posture as you are cutting vegetables.

Driving

Driving is one of my favorite daily activities to work on my core and postural stability. There are also transitions between static and dynamic postures while driving. You want to ensure you are sitting straight, so adjusting the seat and maintaining an upright posture with good lumbar support is step number one. Notice how this improves any back or neck discomfort you may feel while driving. Notice how you can turn your neck to see next to you or behind you more easily in a good posture than in a non-optimal posture.

While stopped at a light, use it as an opportunity to make any minor corrections in your posture and to focus on your diaphragmatic belly breathing. A few minutes of focusing on your breathing is much better than looking at your phone. The only problem is that you may be so mindful and relaxed that you still don't realize the light turned green.

Turning a corner is another excellent time to increase your awareness of postural stability. The next time you go to make a turn, engage that core by creating some intra-abdominal pressure. Notice how stable your body feels taking that turn with some awareness of your postural and spinal stability compared to not focusing on it.

Summary for Daily Life Activities

Paying attention to how you do even the most mundane daily tasks can be the foundation for building your postural and spinal stability. The times you can bring awareness through these daily activities will help you transition the feeling from conscious to subconscious. When you get to that point, you will notice that you are automatically doing things with ideal quality of coordination and movement. You will catch yourself doing things in a non-optimal way without much conscious effort. That is an excellent place to be.

Exercise & Sports

Exercise and sports are among the most problematic activities for people with postural and spinal instability, simply because it's much easier to overdo them. This is true whether it's resuming a weight training regimen, starting a new exercise routine you were not conditioned for, or getting back to full participation in a sport. I regularly see patients' neck and back symptoms flare up after participating in exercise or sports. Once we start addressing the root problem of their postural and spinal instability, I've seen the prevalence of these exacerbations considerably diminish.

It is an art to know when to go back to your exercise or sport and how to modify your routine to accommodate, but it ultimately comes down to competence. First, you must practice balance and stability with less demanding positions. Once you can complete the exercises while lying on your back with your legs supported, you can move on to more challenging activities. Eventually, you will get to the point where you have the competence and capacity to handle any exercise or sport because you know how to control your alignment, breathing, and intra-abdominal pressure throughout the activity.

For example, in my clinic, after relieving someone's pain and restoring mobility, I start them with postural correction, breathing awareness, and baseline competence of maintaining intra-abdominal pressure in a 3-month supine position. I progress their stability capacity in this position with increasingly demanding mobility and load. Then I pick developmental positions to train their postural and spinal stability relevant to their unique weaknesses and specific requirements of their sport. So, working with a runner, I might focus on crawling, bear walking, and single-leg stability. Or I might concentrate on side plank variations, a split stance squat, and lunge variations for a tennis player. After that, I train stability and strength in dynamic movements specific to the exercise or sport.

To get back to exercising or playing a sport in your own life, you must first spend some time doing this fundamental work. For some, it will take weeks. For others, it could take months. But as your awareness and ability grow, you will be able to do what you need to do during an exercise to maintain postural integrity, correct and maintain good postural alignment through the exercise, maintain steady abdominal breathing during the activity, and maintain adequate intra-abdominal pressure throughout the movement. If you cannot do this, the exercise demands may exceed your ability to control the exercise. Usually, this is due to the activity being too challenging or using too much weight, so you will need to back off and work up to higher levels more gradually.

Let's look at how you can apply these techniques during a few different exercises.

Gluteal Bridge

A gluteal bridge is an exercise that trains the core, gluteal muscles, and hamstrings. Lying on your back with your knees bent and your feet flat on the floor. Raise your hips off the floor, extending your hips and spine towards the sky.

There are several ways to improve this exercise's stability and quality of movement. First, bring your lower rib cage down to create a parallel position with your pelvis. Then engage your stability 360 degrees around your trunk. Then raise your hips while maintaining the alignment, not overextending your back, which loses the rib cage and pelvis parallel alignment, while maintaining intra-abdominal pressure and a steady diaphragmatic breathing pattern.

Push-Up

A push-up is a typical upper body strengthening exercise. It trains the core, chest, shoulder, and triceps muscles. A push-up is performed on your stomach with your hands under your shoulders. Push into the ground with your hands, press your body away from the ground, and return to the starting position.

To improve the stability and quality of movement in this exercise, you can do the following: Start in a plank position on your hands (the top of the push-up position) and correct your postural alignment in this position, keeping your ribs down, chest open, shoulders back and down, and neck long. Your hips should be in line with your trunk, not sagging towards the ground, causing an arch in the back, or hiked towards the sky, causing a rounding out of your back. Ensure good arm support by spreading your fingers, flattening your palms, and turning your elbow creases to face forward. Then you would maintain intra-abdominal pressure 360 degrees around and keep steady breathing while you progress through each repetition, correcting your alignment each time.

If you cannot maintain all of that, the exercise is too challenging and needs to be modified. In the case of the push-up, you could do a push-up on your knees or an incline push-up on a bench or table. If that is still too difficult, you could start getting more stable and robust with a plank position on your hands and progress to a push-up over time.

Squat

A squat is another common bodyweight exercise, though some people avoid it like the plague. They are too worried that they may injure themselves, perhaps because someone in the medical field told them that squatting is dangerous. It is not—if you do it correctly. A squat movement trains the core and strengthens the hip and knee extensors. Standing shoulder-width apart, squat down, lowering your bottom towards the ground, and then stand back up.

The squat is a more challenging movement that requires more attention, especially when it comes to postural alignment. First, pay attention to the support function of the feet. Weight should be in all four corners of the foot, with the arch maintained. Knees should be in line with your feet. Maintain good spinal alignment. Create intra-abdominal pressure, descend by hinging from the hips and bending at the knees to a level you are comfortable with, keeping your weight back on your heels and not allowing your knees to come forward beyond your toes. The key is to maintain the postural alignment of your feet, knees, and spine as you move up and down through the movement. Of course, remember to keep your intra-abdominal pressure and steady breathing.

For many people with poor stability, the spine will collapse (flex) or arch (hyperextend), the foot arch will collapse (flatten), the knees will migrate towards each other, losing the optimal alignment of the knee over the foot, and the knees may come forward beyond the toes.

If a squat is too challenging for you, it may be due to a lack of mobility in your thoracic spine, ankle, hips, or knees, a non-optimal postural and spinal stability, or excessive weight. Modifications could include standing from sitting in a chair, using a hand on a table or chair in front of you for support, or lessening the weight (if you were using any).

Aerobic Exercises

When it comes to aerobic exercises such as jumping rope, riding the elliptical, running, biking, etc., all you need to do is focus on the same principles while going through the motions. The corrections will be more subtle, a straightening of your spine, engagement of the core in line with your demands, and steady nasal diaphragmatic breathing. You will feel more stable, efficient, and robust in your movements if done correctly. It's a beautiful feeling, and some focus on it while exercising will only reinforce this inner strength.

Sports

When it comes to sports, whether soccer, tennis, basketball, golf, etc., you don't want to be thinking of any of this while you are playing; you may be aware of your alignment or your breathing, but there is no time to be conscious of these fine details while engaged in sport. You need to get to the point of unconscious competence. You can do that by working on the principles and exercises discussed in this book. Then your sports participation will improve with less injury and pain risk.

Conclusion

Going to a gym hurts my soul. I find myself observing how people are moving and exercising. I can't help it; I'm a PT. Most people I see in the gym exercise with poor alignment, poor breathing patterns, and poor stability. I also see less than ideal form, uncontrolled movements that are short and quick, and weight that is too heavy to control. It pains me because I know that people are setting themselves up to fail, wear down their bodies, and possibly injure themselves.

It can be challenging to think about all this while exercising, but it is safer. You can improve the quality, stability, and integrity of your workouts, building real functional strength and giving you the best chance of preventing injury or pain in the future.

CHAPTER 9

Getting Additional Help

What Are Your Options?

Have you been suffering from chronic neck and back pain for years? Have you thought that time would take care of it? Have you visited many physicians looking for a diagnosis? Have you tried multiple interventions or relied on painkillers? You're not alone. Millions of people have dealt with the same problems and fallen into the same trap. I hope that you now realize the solution to your neck or back problem is not a quick fix but is more complex than most health care professionals make it out to be.

If you have suffered chronic neck and back pain for years, you have probably altered your life to accommodate your spine problem. You likely stopped exercising or doing things you enjoy because of your spine problem. Maybe you have even stopped living the life you want to live because of your spine problem.

I hope this book has given you a better understanding of why you have been dealing with your spine problem for so long. I also hope that it has given you a possible solution to your problem. I hope that this book has given you—**HOPE**.

We all know the popular definition of insanity—*doing the same thing and expecting a different outcome.* If you are stuck in this place, get out! Don't keep spinning your wheels with the same failed interventions, and don't believe there is nothing you can do but accept the pain and limitations. You are wasting your precious time, energy, and money. You are wasting your life.

No matter how long you have been dealing with this problem, the only way it will change is to **ACT**. Start with these simple things:

- Write out your 'health timeline'
- Take pictures of your posture
- Learn how to correct your posture
- Practice the breathing exercises
- Try the stabilization exercises
- Be more mindful in your everyday life

You will likely feel better if you follow the tips outlined in this book. That may make all the difference for some, and I hope that is true for you.

But for others, it might take a little more help. If that's you, what are your options?

Why Painkillers, Injections, and Surgery Are Not Great Options

Let's start with what you should not do. Don't rely on painkillers or injections to get by. And you don't need spinal surgery unless you have significant spinal column integrity problems or neurological compromise. It is perfectly understandable if you've already had surgery or are using pain medications to help, but wouldn't you rather get to a point where you don't need more surgeries and don't have to rely on medicines for the rest of your life?

Although pain killers and injections may give some relief, they have disadvantages. They can have lasting side effects. They merely mask the pain rather than address the root cause of the problem. The relief may only last a few hours, and you can become reliant on them for months or years. They can give you a false sense of security, making you believe that you are doing okay because you can't feel any problems, only to get blindsided by another flare-up.

There is a time and place for medications, especially in acute situations. But they should not be used to cover up the need to address the root cause of the problem and should not be taken casually. Our reliance on pain medications to treat spine pain has contributed to the national opioid crisis, resulting in the suffering and death of millions of Americans. I strongly encourage you to find other means of addressing your pain and spine problems that are less addicting and potentially harmful to your health.

And what about spine surgery? I spoke in Chapter 2 about the different kinds of spine surgeries and their indications. They are a solution for many when done at the right time for the right reasons, but spinal surgery also has many disadvantages. For one, they are expensive. Then there are the possible immediate risks, including a reaction to anesthesia or other drugs, bleeding, infection, blood clots, stroke, heart attack, and nerve damage. The specific surgery chosen may not address the underlying root cause of your problem. And the trauma of the surgery itself may adversely affect your muscles and fascia, affecting your ability to function and move properly, especially when patients are not getting routine physical therapy after surgery. It may further sensitize your pain sensitivity problem. A spinal fusion (which fuses two or more vertebrae) may potentially wear down levels above and below the fusion, resulting in possible issues down the road.

As with medication, there is a time and place for spinal surgery, mainly when neurological compromise has caused muscle weakness, severe spinal trauma has led to spinal fractures, or significant instability has left the spinal cord potentially compromised. But the truth is that spine surgery is overutilized, especially in the US. The stats speak for themselves. Spinal surgery is not a good solution for the type of everyday spinal instability I most often see in my patients, which we have discussed in this book.

What Else Can You Do?

You can take what you have learned and try to strengthen yourself independently. You can work with a personal trainer to work on your core. Be sure to find one that is right for you, someone who has some knowledge of the principles in this book. You can work with a massage therapist or a bodyworker to address your muscle imbalances and fascial restrictions but remember that addresses only one part of the equation (the flexibility and mobility, not the stability and strength). You can take a group exercise class, but that may not be specific enough to address your stability issue. You can see an acupuncturist, but that would most likely address the pain and energetic influences rather than the underlying stability issue. You can practice Yoga or work with a Pilates instructor but remember that the quality of the postural stability through those poses and exercises is more important than the philosophy behind them. You can see a physical therapist or a chiropractor but find someone who is going to address the underlying issues, not one who is just going to slap electrical stimulation pads and a hot pack on, do little hands-on work, and have you go through routine rehab exercises on your own with little supervision.

I support everything above and occasionally use these interventions to help with my issues. But I don't rely on them, and I don't expect them to solve my spinal stability issues. Interventions not focused on addressing the underlying stability problem will not get you to where you want to go. Even interventions geared toward stability may have the right intention but fall short in execution or may even be harmful if not done correctly. Pulling your belly button to your spine in your Pilates class is problematic and will not engage your core correctly. Doing core work on your own or in an exercise class that is too advanced will only reinforce your compensations and muscle imbalances.

I have treated hundreds of spine cases over more than 20 years, so I know the pitfalls of well-meaning approaches that either don't help or don't address an underlying stability issue. Pilates, yoga, personal training, and group classes can be helpful, but it often depends on the patient's unique history and physical capacity. On the other hand, physical therapy could be the right help based on your personal needs and goals, using methods proven to address the actual root causes of pain and dysfunction.

Why Choose Physical Therapy?

Physical Therapy is a dynamic profession with an established theoretical and scientific base that uses widespread clinical applications and treatments to restore, maintain, and promote optimal physical function.

Physical Therapists:

- Diagnose and manage movement dysfunction to enhance physical and functional abilities.

- Restore, maintain, and promote optimal physical function, wellness, fitness, and quality of life related to movement and health.

- Prevent the onset, symptoms, and progression of impairments, functional limitations, and disabilities resulting from diseases, disorders, conditions, or injuries.

Physical therapists engage in an examination process that includes taking history, conducting a systems review, and performing tests and measures to identify potential and existing problems. Physical therapists establish a diagnosis, prognosis, and plan of care by performing evaluations, synthesizing the examination data, and determining whether the issues to be addressed are within the scope of the physical therapist's practice. Based on their judgments about diagnosis, prognosis, and patient goals; physical therapists provide interventions, conduct reexaminations, modify interventions as necessary to achieve anticipated goals and expected outcomes, and develop and implement discharge plans.

So why is physical therapy best suited for spine problems, especially stability problems?

First, a person's history is a significant factor when evaluating a spine problem. Our unique history inquiry of past surgeries, injuries, and traumas is an essential piece of the puzzle. A physical therapist is trained to take a good history, and we often have more time than doctors to take one. Taking a good history is one of the hallmarks of our evaluation process and, in my opinion, the most crucial part.

Second, the flexibility and mobility of muscles is a critical aspect of the equation in postural muscle imbalances. So alleviating spine problems often requires your muscles to be stretched and the joints to be mobilized. Physical therapy is focused explicitly on restoring muscle flexibility and joint mobility.

Third, postural awareness and the ability to correct your posture are vital when addressing spinal issues. You need to understand your specific postural makeup and how to improve upon it through postural corrective exercises. Postural correction and retraining are also hallmarks of physical therapy.

Fourth, the muscular system's stability and strength must also be addressed for most spinal conditions. That is the other side of the equation in postural muscle imbalances. For it to work, you must be specific about what areas of the body are stabilized or strengthened instead of a generic core or muscle-strengthening approach. Physical therapy is specifically suited to restore stability and strength where you need it.

Lastly, coordination training is critical to integrating the restored flexibility, mobility, stability, and strength. Learning (or re-learning) how to move is necessary for maintaining your gains. Otherwise, falling back to old, non-optimal movement patterns is easy. Physical therapy is uniquely qualified to help people learn to move in a more coordinated and efficient way.

Physical therapy is well suited to address all the various impairments involved with spinal conditions, not just one piece of this very complex puzzle. The educational training in anatomy, physiology, neurology, medical pathology, biomechanics, kinesiology, manual therapy, modalities, exercise prescription, and behavioral psychology is a well-rounded basis for addressing a total-body problem. A massage therapist may be better at soft tissue work, or a chiropractor may be an expert in manipulating the spine. Still, no other health care professional is better suited for addressing all the different aspects of the body's ability to move well than a physical therapist is.

How to Choose a Physical Therapist

When choosing a physical therapist, you could ask your doctor, do an online search, check with your insurance company, or get a recommendation from friends. If you aren't familiar with physical therapy, you are likely to choose a clinic based on location, hours of operation, and whether they take your insurance or not. These are factors. Therapy can't help if you aren't able to go to it. But an excellent location and good hours do not ensure you will get the help you need from a person you can trust, nor does a recommendation from a doctor who may never have even been to the clinic. To get the best care, you want to look for certain qualities and practices that set them apart from the average practitioner. Choosing a physical therapist is a personal decision, so take the time to evaluate the person or clinic you will have to trust with your health and life.

Here are some things to look for:

One-on-One Care

There are many different types of outpatient physical therapy practices and clinics. Some are large regional and national entities with multiple locations, some are small practices, and some are solo practitioners.

You may find the right therapist at any of them. How much one-on-one time the therapist will spend with you is crucial. The more one-on-one time you have with your therapist, the greater the therapist's chances of having the time, energy, and freedom to help you. Many clinics may say they provide one-on-one care, but then you only get to see the therapist for a short time before being told to do exercises on your own or with an assistant. To get an idea of what your experience will be like, ask the clinic how many patients the therapist sees in an hour. If they see more than one patient during your visit, it's not exactly one-on-one care, is it?

Manual Therapy Approach

I recommend a physical therapist with specialized manual therapy training. A physical therapist with manual therapy experience or credentials is likely to be, though not always, a better therapist.

Why? Because they work on developing their hands-on skills. Manual therapy techniques are intended to improve tissue extensibility, increase range of motion, induce relaxation, mobilize or manipulate soft tissues and joints, modulate pain, and reduce swelling, inflammation, or restriction. Manual therapy techniques include joint mobilization/manipulation, dry needling, functional mobilization, neural mobilization, soft tissue mobilization, myofascial release, friction massage, passive range of motion, and manual traction.

Also, physical therapists with manual therapy training tend to have better clinical reasoning skills. Because they must think through how to solve problems with their hands, they can get to the root cause and connect how other body issues may contribute to the symptoms or limitations. Many therapists will develop some of this through experience, but manual therapy programs and courses focus on teaching these higher-level clinical reasoning skills.

As with other health care professionals, physical therapists graduate with basic education (if you consider the 6-7 years of undergraduate and graduate education basic). After that, it is on the physical therapist as a professional to expand upon that education through continuing education courses, mentorship, clinical experience, and research. While experience always helps, time in the profession alone isn't enough to develop the necessary skills and knowledge.

So, whether the physical therapist is a recent grad or a seasoned practitioner, work with someone dedicated to continuous learning and improvement. An outpatient physical therapist with a manual therapy certification is most likely committed to doing so. They will have a better arsenal of tools in their toolkit, and are more likely to have a clinical-reasoned approach rather than a protocol-based approach, which means they can deliver better outcomes in a shorter period.

Holistic Approach

Look for a therapist or clinic that offers a holistic approach to their care. You want someone who will treat you as a person, not the condition or complaint you call them about. They should address you as a unique individual with a need or a set of physical problems. Everyone is different when it comes to background, history, and capabilities. No two disc herniation patients are the same and should not be treated similarly. It would be best if you got personalized care suited to your specific needs and desires.

A clinic with a holistic approach will be good listeners during their initial phone conversation and the history-taking process. They will take the time to get to know you before beginning treatment. They will ask you about your goals and the outcome that you want. They will be curious about your personal life. They will ask you how your condition has affected your life.

When you receive care from a clinician that considers your mind, body, and spirit, you will have a better chance of getting the desired outcome. And it will be a more enjoyable and meaningful experience in the process.

Experience and Specialized Training

You want to find a clinic that has specific experience and training in treating the condition or problem that you may have. Clinical experience is important, and you should be able to take comfort in knowing that a therapist has dealt with issues and problems like yours. You want to know they can deliver actual results. So, make sure you ask them. Be specific about your situation and your needs.

In general, look for therapists who have specialized training in dry needling. Dry needling is the most effective and efficient way to address the muscular and fascia aspect of spine problems. Finding one therapist who can do it all will save you time than finding a different place to go for dry needling alone. And they will likely be able to address any pain resulting from the muscle dysfunction quickly and thoroughly, restoring normal muscle tone, balance, coordination, and strength.

For spinal and spine stability conditions specifically, look for a clinician with specialized training in breathing dysfunction, global postural approach, or spinal stability, especially those with **Dynamic Neuromuscular Stabilization (DNS)** training. You can check this website for a list of DNS Certified Practitioners (htttps://www.rehabps.cz/rehab/certified_practitioners) and DNS Certified Exercise Trainers (htttps://www.rehabps.cz/rehab/certified_trainers).

In-Network versus Out-of-Network

Ideally, the best clinic would be in-network with your insurance, but don't limit yourself to only the clinics on some insurance company's list. The best therapist for your needs may be part of a different network. Often, they will not be a part of any network because the problem with taking the insurance company's money is that you must follow the insurance company's rules.

Many personalized therapy clinics do not take insurance because they would not be able to provide the same quality and level of care under insurance that they can independently. This means they aren't bogged down with the relentless work required to maintain a busy volume-based, in-network practice. They will likely have more time and energy to get to the root of the problem and address it. Out-of-network therapists may seem more expensive at first because you pay more out of pocket, but the value and long-term health benefits will far outweigh the cost if you get lasting relief in fewer sessions and don't have to keep coming back for the same problem. They also may be harder to get in to see because they are highly sought after for their quality and personalization. I wish this wasn't the case, but it has become the reality of our healthcare system.

Conclusion

You are not likely to find a physical therapist or chiropractor who has all these qualifications and meets all these standards. But if you find a clinic or therapist who meets some or most of what I have outlined, you can feel confident trusting them to help you solve your neck or back problems.

CHAPTER 10

Moving Forward

Moving Forward

Wherever you find yourself in your journey to overcome chronic neck or back pain, I hope this book has been informative and helpful. For some, this book may be all that is necessary to get back on track, but others may need additional help. I'm here to assist you in any way that I can. Here are some of the different ways I can be of service.

I have **free guides** on my website if you are unsure what to do about your neck and back problems. They are for people who are just starting to have problems or want to learn what they can do about their problems independently. They are full of helpful information to figure out what the next steps might be.

If you have been dealing with your problem for quite some time, failed other interventions, did the research, and would like to speak with me directly about your situation, I would be happy to set up a **Phone Consult** or a **Discovery Session**. This allows you to give me an overview of your problems, what's worked, what hasn't worked, and find out what could be done. The Discovery Session is a free 30-minute in-person or online session, allowing you to meet me directly. If you know you want to avoid long-term suffering and future exacerbations of your spine issue, or if you want a second opinion about your problem, the Phone Consult or Discovery Session is your best bet.

I'm available for one-on-one **In-Person Sessions** at one of my two practice locations in Bethesda or Olney, Maryland. I am also available for **Telehealth Sessions** and have seen remarkable success in helping people through their neck and back problems online.

Final Thoughts

When I decided to write a book that could help people live healthier, happier lives based on my years of knowledge and clinical experience, I took some time before deciding on what subject to write about. I could have written about many other subjects. I contemplated a book on self-management of pain, headaches, the benefits of dry needling, or the benefits of manual therapy.

But I knew I wanted to write a book to help people suffering from spine problems. Spine problems are incredibly prevalent. Neck and back cases make up most of my schedule, and spine health is fundamental to overall body and movement health, so I knew that it could also help anyone who was dealing with pain, postural problems, or movement problems, even if they didn't suffer from neck and back pain.

I also knew that this book might be read by other health practitioners, fitness trainers, and health coaches who come across clients who deal with these spinal problems. I wanted to educate them on what I have learned so that they can potentially have a more significant impact on the people they serve.

It didn't take long before I decided I wanted to write about—**STABILITY**. I'm passionate about addressing the real problem. Everything else I contemplated wouldn't address the real problem, merely the symptoms of an underlying problem. I have seen this with my spinal issues and those of hundreds of patients.

Underlying postural stability is the root cause of many people's spine problems, but it's not commonly recognized or appropriately addressed. I am a truth seeker by nature. When I realized the truth of how postural stability is the basis of how we were meant to move and is the best antidote to the degradation of our spine and body, I had to share it. I talk about it daily with my patients, my colleague physical therapists, and other health and fitness professionals.

Addressing your muscle imbalances, restoring your optimal breath, and improving your postural and dynamic stability is the answer for many of us. Whether it's a baby with developmental delays, a child with coordination issues, a middle-aged person with neck and back pain, or an older adult suffering from degenerative spine disorders, improving your postural stability is the basis for addressing all these problems from a fundamental place. It all starts with foundational spinal and postural stability.

My hope for anyone who reads this book is that it opens your eyes to what is possible and that you experience change through this postural stability work on your own. I don't want you to believe what I'm saying because I have written it here. I want you to experience it and verify it is true. Discover the gift of breath and postural stability inherent in you since you were a baby. If you do this, you will feel better, move better, and be a better version of yourself. You will become stronger—from the inside out.

Be Well!

Tamer

Resources

Book Resources:

www.freedomfromneckandbackpain.com

Issa Physical Therapy & Wellness:

www.issaptwellness.com

Set Up a Phone Consult:

https://www.issaptwellness.com/Talk-to-a-PT-on-the-Phone/a~17650/article.html

Set Up a Discovery Session:

https://www.issaptwellness.com/Free-Discovery-Visit/a~17651/article.html

About the Author

Dr. Tamer Issa, PT, DPT

Dr. Issa founded Issa Physical Therapy in 2005 to provide the highest quality physical therapy care in the Washington, DC Metro area. The cornerstone of the practice is a holistic approach to care that aims to treat the person, not just the physical problem. He seeks to help people feel, move, and live better without relying on medications, injections, and surgery.

Dr. Issa earned his Bachelor of Physiotherapy degree from Saxion University Enschede in the Netherlands and his Doctor of Physical Therapy Degree from the University of St. Augustine. He credits this early education, ongoing continuing education, clinical experience, and clinical teaching experience for giving him the knowledge and skills to effectively diagnose, treat, and prevent neuromusculoskeletal problems.

Dr. Issa's clinical expertise includes myofascial trigger point therapy, trigger point dry needling, orthopedic manual therapy, headaches, craniomandibular (TMJ) dysfunction, scoliosis, and other spinal conditions. He has a particular interest and advanced training in a global approach to postural dysfunction, breathing dysfunction, postural and spinal stability, motor control, and functional stability and strength.

Dr. Issa strongly believes that only through an individualized one-on-one care model can clinicians accurately diagnose, identify the underlying sources, and comprehensively address the problem. This approach leads to faster pain relief in fewer visits and preventing episodic recurrences that are all too common.

For these reasons, so many people have sought out Issa Physical Therapy & Wellness for a holistic approach to their care that is aimed at not just treating symptoms but getting them back to living their life to the fullest.

During his free time, Dr. Issa enjoys spending time with his family and friends, cooking, hiking, playing golf, fishing, and learning new ways to better himself.

Education:

- Doctor of Physical Therapy (DPT) degree from the University of St. Augustine for Health Sciences in 2006
- B.S. degree in Physiotherapy from the Saxion Hogeschool Enschede in the Netherlands in 1998
- B.S. degree in Exercise and Sport Science from Pennsylvania State University in 1995

Certifications:

- Board-Certified Clinical Specialist in Orthopedic Physical Therapy (OCS) by the American Physical Therapy Association
- Certified Orthopedic Manipulative Therapist (COMT) by the North American Institute of Orthopedic Manual Therapy (NAIOMT)

- Dynamic Neuromuscular Stabilization (DNS) Certified Practitioner from the Rehabilitation Prague School
- Certified in Manual Trigger Point Therapy and Needling by the Dr. Janet Travell Seminar Series (now known as Myopain Seminars)
- Certified in Functional Dry Needling by Kinetacore (now known as Evidence in Motion)
- Titleist Performance Institute (TPI) Certified- Level I

www.ingramcontent.com/pod-product-compliance
Lightning Source LLC
Chambersburg PA
CBHW071351210526
45465CB00001B/55